Handy
DIET and
NUTRITION
Guide

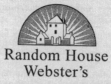

Random House
Webster's

Handy
DIET and
NUTRITION
Guide

RANDOM HOUSE
NEW YORK

Trademarks

A number of entered words that we have reason to believe constitute trademarks have been designated as such. However, no attempt has been made to designate as trademarks or service marks all terms or words in which proprietary rights might exist. The inclusion, exclusion, or definition of a word or term is not intended to affect, or to express a judgment on, the validity or legal status of the word or term as a trademark, service mark, or other proprietary term.

Acknowledgment

We would like to thank all who helped produce this edition. The expert advice and contributions of Ellen Liskov, R.D., M.P.H., Ambulatory Nutrition Specialist at Yale-New Haven Hospital, New Haven, Connecticut, were invaluable. As adviser to the book, Ms. Liskov readily shared her expertise in nutrition, particularly in planning the Basic Healthy Diet, Basic Weight Loss, and Special Diets Sections.

Special thanks go also to Ilene Duchin, for revision and updating of the Composition of Foods section.

Contents

A Word About Nutrition, Health, and Diet

The importance of proper nutrition is universally recognized. It is well established that nutritional factors play a role in at least five of the ten leading causes of death in the United States, including coronary heart disease, stroke, diabetes, certain forms of cancer, and atherosclerosis. The debate over exactly what constitutes a "healthy" diet continues as further discoveries are made almost daily about various nutritional components and well-being. Unfortunately, in recent years, the public has received too many conflicting reports regarding food, nutrition, and health, which has led to confusion and skepticism. Overall, however, the quest for health and wellness has prompted many people to improve their eating habits, exercise regularly, and control their weight.

The purpose of *Eat Smart* is to offer some general guidelines for formulating a diet that is nutritionally sound for most healthy people and to suggest ways to meet special needs associated with certain health problems. The fundamentals of a healthy diet are described and a 7-day meal plan for sensible eating is provided. This same meal plan is also adjusted for a basic weight-loss program of 1,800 or 1,200 calories per day. In addition, there are outlines for diets that alter the amount of sodium, fats, carbohydrate, fiber, lactose, purines, and calcium consumed. Suggestions are made for ensuring the nutritional adequacy of a vegetarian diet. The information provided in this book is built upon the most current and strongest scientific findings available.

This second edition of *Eat Smart* supplements the diets with information on the Recommended Daily Allowances for vitamins and minerals as well as good food sources for particular nutrients, height and weight standards, calculation of calorie and fat requirements, estimates of calories burned with exercise, how to read a food label, and healthy cooking techniques. The Composition of Foods table covers more than 1,000 separate foods, listing the key nutritional data for a serving of each: calories, protein, fat (total and saturated), cholesterol, carbohydrate (total and fiber), and sodium. This information allows consumers to evaluate the foods being eaten and to develop meal plans based on the guidelines offered in each specific diet.

Nutritional needs are like fingerprints; no two are alike. It is impossible to develop a diet that is perfectly balanced for every individual because nutritional needs are influenced by a variety of factors, including age, sex, body size, activity level, metabolism, medication usage, medical history and health status, and genetic predisposition to various diseases. Therefore, discuss your unique nutritional requirements with a health care provider before beginning any type of diet or regimen. A registered dietitian (R.D.) can help develop an eating plan for good health and wellness.

BASIC HEALTHY DIET

Dietary Guidelines for Americans

The Dietary Guidelines for Americans were revised in 1990 by the U.S. Department of Agriculture and the U.S. Department of Health and Human Services. They reflect the understanding that many common illnesses in American society are related to a diet that is excessive in calories, fat, saturated fat, cholesterol, sodium, and sugar and that lacks complex carbohydrate and fiber. In addition, recommendations are made to define "moderation" in the consumption of alcoholic beverages. While diseases of nutritional deficiency are quite uncommon (in fact many Americans are "overnourished"), some people may not be obtaining an optimal amount of iron and calcium from their diet.

To stay healthy:

1. Eat a variety of foods

In order to obtain the more than 40 different nutrients essential for good health, choose a variety of foods from each of the food groups in the Food Guide Pyramid (page 6). No one food or food group can provide all the nutrients needed by the body.

2. Maintain a healthy weight

The risk of many illnesses such as high blood pressure, heart disease, stroke, adult-onset diabetes, and certain types of cancer is increased in people who are overweight and have too much body fat. Refer to the chart on page 227 to determine if your weight, based upon your age and height, is within a healthy range. The weights at the upper end of the range are most appropriate for muscular or large-boned individuals (usually men) while the lower end is best suited for smaller-boned people. The health risks mentioned above are associated with too much body fat, not weight from muscle and bone mass. This is particularly true in "apple-shaped" people who tend to accumulate excess fat in the abdomen as opposed to "pear-shaped" people who carry excess weight in their thighs and buttocks. An easy method to determine if you have too much abdominal fat is to calculate your waist-to-hip ratio. To do this, stand relaxed and measure your waist near your navel, where it is smallest, and then your hips, over the buttocks, where they are largest. Divide your waist measurement by your hips measurement and if the number is near or over 1.0, it means that you probably have too much abdominal fat. Weight-loss diets are discussed in further detail on pages 26–38.

Although many people aim to be thin, there is no health benefit to weighing much less than the lowest weight in the range. In fact, the risk of certain diseases, such as osteoporosis, is increased in individuals who are too thin. Extreme underweight may be suggestive of anorexia nervosa or other health problems. Always report any sudden weight loss to your doctor.

3. Choose a diet low in fat, saturated fat, and cholesterol

A diet low in fat may reduce the risk of many illnesses, including heart disease, some forms of cancer, and obesity. Too much saturated fat or dietary cholesterol can raise blood cholesterol levels, a strong risk factor for heart disease. Saturated fat is found in most animal products, tropical oils such as coconut and palm oil, cocoa butter, and hydrogenated (solid) vegetable fats. Fish, chicken, and 1% fat or skim milk dairy products have less saturated fat than red meat or higher-fat dairy products. Dietary cholesterol is found only in animal foods, especially eggs and organ meats. In addition to limiting organ meats and eggs, keep serving sizes of meat, poultry, or fish to about 6 ounces daily (the size of two decks of cards). Other types of fat include polyunsaturated (found in corn, safflower, sunflower, and soybean oils) and monounsaturated (abundant in olive oil, canola oil, and nuts). Use polyunsaturated or monounsaturated fats instead of saturated fats whenever possible. Other suggestions for heart healthy eating can be found on pages 42–45.

A healthy diet should contain no more than 30% calories from total fat, 10% from saturated fat, and 300 milligrams of cholesterol. The actual amount of fat and saturated fat to be eaten per day can be determined from the calorie needs.

EXAMPLE: 2,000 calories needed a day
2,000 calories × 0.30 = 600 fat calories
2,000 calories × 0.10 = 200 saturated fat calories

After calculating the calories allowed from both fat and saturated fat, divide each number by 9 (the number of calories per gram of fat) to get a daily allowance in grams.

EXAMPLE: 600 fat calories ÷ 9 = 67 grams total fat
200 saturated fat calories ÷ 9 = 22 grams saturated fat

4. Choose a diet with plenty of vegetables, fruits, and grain products

Fiber, the indigestible portion of foods, is important for bowel regularity and is also a factor in the prevention of constipation, diverticular disease, and certain forms of cancer. The majority of foods from the vegetable, fruit, bread, cereal, rice, and pasta groups are naturally low in fat content and are good sources of complex carbohydrate and fiber. By emphasizing these food groups in the diet, as the Food Guide Pyramid suggests, most people can boost their fiber intake and limit fats at the same time. Refer to the High-Fiber Diet (page 45) for more information.

5. Use sugars only in moderation

The term "sugar" includes more than just white or brown granulated sugar. Other sugars are honey, maple syrup, corn syrup, molasses, fructose (fruit sugar), maltose (grain sugar), and lactose (milk sugar). A diet high in sugar content, especially when sugars are eaten frequently between meals or are in a sticky form, increases the risk of tooth decay. Aside from the fruit, grain, or milk sugars listed above, the others do not provide a significant source of nutrients—only calories. To cut calories without sacrificing essential nutrients, reduce the intake of "empty calorie" sources of sugar like regular soft drinks and candy.

6. Use salt and sodium only in moderation

Most Americans consume far more sodium than is required for good health. A high-sodium diet may increase the likelihood of developing high blood pressure, a strong risk factor for both heart disease and stroke. Individuals with high blood pressure can often lower it by restricting their intake of sodium, losing excess weight, limiting alcohol, and exercising regularly. Most health authorities agree that a healthy diet should contain no more than 3,000 milligrams (mg) of sodium a day, and some say 2,400 milligrams is more appropriate. Major sources of sodium in the American diet are table salt (1 teaspoon has 2,300 mg of sodium); condiments such as soy sauce, teriyaki or barbecue sauce, pickles, olives, catsup, and mustard; canned foods; snack foods; cured or processed meat, poultry, and fish; and convenience foods, including frozen dinners and flavored rice, stuffing, potato, or pasta mixes. For further information, refer to the Low-Sodium Diet (page 39).

7. If you drink alcoholic beverages, do so in moderation

Alcoholic beverages contribute calories to the diet but basically no other nutrients. Too much alcohol in the diet may lead to nutritional inadequacies because alcohol can replace more nutritious foods and because vitamins and minerals may not be as well absorbed by the body. In addition, excessive alcohol intake can also lead to diseases of the liver, pancreas, brain, and heart. While recent health reports have indicated that moderate alcohol consumption may decrease the risk of heart disease, this has not been conclusively established. If you do choose to drink, follow the guidelines below. Moderation is defined as no more than one drink a day for women and two drinks a day for men. One drink is equal to one 12-ounce regular beer, 5 ounces of wine, or 1½ ounces of hard liquor (80 proof).

A seven-day menu plan, which incorporates the principles of the Dietary Guidelines for Americans, can be found on pages 20–25.

The Food Guide Pyramid

The Food Guide Pyramid was developed to help Americans achieve a balanced diet through an understanding of what to eat and how much to eat from each food group. The model shows which foods should be emphasized and which should be consumed in relatively lesser quantities in order to implement the Dietary Guidelines for Americans. Each food group is important because it contributes some of the nutrients needed for good health.

At the base of the pyramid is the bread, cereal, rice, and pasta group. In order to maintain a diet low in fat, high in complex carbohydrate and fiber, and full of many different vitamins and minerals, the

Fats, Oils, and Sweets
USE SPARINGLY

Milk Group

Meat Group

2-3 SERVINGS

2-3 SERVINGS

Vegetable Group

Fruit Group

3-5 SERVINGS

2-4 SERVINGS

Bread Group

6-11 SERVINGS

highest number of servings per day should be from this group. These foods are not fattening if the right selections are made and portion sizes are monitored. This includes using only a small amount of added fats and sugars in their preparation or as spreads and limiting most baked goods, such as cakes, cookies, doughnuts, pastries, and pies. Whenever possible, choose whole wheat bread and whole grain cereals for their higher fiber content.

Count one serving as: 1 slice bread; ½ bagel; hamburger roll or English muffin; 1 oz. cold cereal; ½ cup cooked hot cereal, rice, or pasta; 1 tortilla; or 1 pancake.

The next level encompasses the vegetable and fruit groups, which are excellent sources of fiber and of vitamins and minerals and generally have low calorie and fat contents. Serve and prepare vegetables with a minimum of butter, margarine, oil, sauce, or salad dressing (count these additions as fat). Whole fruits usually have more fiber than fruit juice. To keep sugar content low, use 100% fruit juice instead of punch, fruit-flavored drinks, or soda (which count as sweets) and purchase canned fruits in their own juice.

Count one serving as: Vegetables: 1 cup raw leafy vegetables; ½ cup cooked or raw other vegetables; ¾ cup vegetable juice; small baked potato.
Fruits: 1 medium piece whole fruit; ½ cup raw or canned fruit; ¾ cup 100% fruit juice.

Many people are surprised to learn that they do not need as much meat, poultry, fish, dry beans and peas, and eggs and nuts as they thought. While these foods do supply protein, iron, zinc, and B vitamins, the animal foods from this group are high in saturated fat and cholesterol. It is best to eat skinless poultry and fish and use lean cuts of red meats such as flank, round or sirloin steak, extra-lean ground beef, center loin or tenderloin pork, and leg of lamb or loin chops. Trim all visible fat and avoid frying. Eat organ meats infrequently and limit egg yolks to 3–4 a week. Use dry beans and peas as an entree for maximum fiber and no saturated fat or cholesterol. Use nuts and seeds in moderation because of their high fat content. In total, about 5–7 ounces a day of cooked meat, poultry, or fish is appropriate.

Count one serving as: 2–3 ounces cooked lean meat, poultry, fish, or
                     seafood (deck of cards size).
                        1 oz. is equal to: 1 egg; 2 Tbsp. peanut butter;
                     ⅓ cup nuts; or ½ cup cooked dry beans or
                     peas.

Foods from the milk, yogurt, and cheese group are important for
providing adequate calcium. Because these foods can supply a lot of
fat, especially saturated fat, choose 1% fat or nonfat milk and yogurt
and low-fat or "part skim" cheeses. Cottage cheese is lower in calcium
than most other cheese. Ice cream and lower-fat alternatives, such as
ice milk or frozen yogurt, contain more sugar but less calcium than
most of the other choices in this group.

Count one serving as: 1 cup milk or yogurt; 2 ounces processed
                     cheese; 1½ ounces natural cheese; or ½ cup
                     ricotta cheese.
                    Count ½ serving as: ½ cup frozen yogurt; ¾ cup
                     ice cream or ice milk; 1 cup cottage cheese.

Fats and sweets are at the top of the pyramid to emphasize that
only a small amount of added fat (butter, margarine, mayonnaise,
salad dressing, oils) and sugar (table sugar, maple syrup, jam and jelly,
corn syrup, honey) is desirable. Too much fat promotes illness, and
sugars can be sources of non-nutritious calories. The amount that can
be used of either depends upon a person's calorie needs to maintain an
ideal weight and fat allowance. When a fat is used, limit saturated
sources such as butter, palm or coconut oils in packaged foods, cocoa
butter, and hydrogenated (solid) shortening.

Reading Food Labels

The Food and Drug Administration requires by law that nearly all
processed foods have a "Nutrition Facts" panel on their packaging.
This standard format allows one to identify the exact content of many
nutrients and to better understand how to fit that food into an overall
diet. Here are some important points about food labeling.

1. Identify the *Serving Size* of the food item. The nutrient content
listed is based on that portion size. If you are going to eat two servings
of that food, you will need to double the numbers shown.

2. The *Nutrient Content* is provided for Calories, Total Fat, Saturated Fat, Cholesterol, Sodium, Total Carbohydrate, Dietary Fiber, Sugar, and Protein. These nutrients were chosen because of their strong link to many diseases afflicting Americans.

3. The *Percentage (%) Daily Value* indicates what portion of the recommended Daily Value is met by one serving of that food item for a person who needs 2,000 calories a day. Based upon calorie needs, one can determine the Daily Value numbers for Total Fat (30% calories), Saturated Fat (10% calories), Carbohydrate (60% calories), and Protein (10% calories). Use the resources in the book as a start or seek the assistance of a registered dietitian. For other nutrients, the Daily Values are the same for everyone, including cholesterol (goal: 300 mg or less daily), sodium (goal: no more than 2,400 mg), and fiber (goal: at least 25 grams a day). In addition, the % Daily Value is provided for vitamins A and C as well as for calcium and iron.

4. If a food product meets certain strict criteria, a *nutrient claim* may appear on the label. The claim gives a general idea of the amount of the nutrient in the product per serving, but it is always best to look at the Nutrition Facts panel for more details. The following terms are allowed:

Free	There is virtually none of the nutrient stated per serving.
Low	The meaning varies for each nutrient. Per serving there can be no more than 140 mg sodium (low sodium); 3 gm total fat (low fat); 1 gm saturated fat (low saturated fat); 20 mg cholesterol (low cholesterol); 40 calories (low calorie).
Very Low	Applies to sodium only. Means no more than 35 mg sodium per serving.
Reduced or less	Contains 25% less of the nutrient stated (fat, sodium, or calories) than the regular version or comparable product.
Light or lite	Contains 50% less fat or sodium or ⅓ less calories than the regular version or comparable product.
% Fat Free	The percent of fat present by weight (not by percent of calories from fat).

Lean	Meat or poultry products containing less than 10 gm fat, 4 gm saturated fat, and 95 mg cholesterol per 3.5 ounce portion (deck of cards size).
Extra Lean	Meat or poultry products containing less than 5 gm fat, 2 gm saturated fat, and 95 mg cholesterol per 3.5 ounce portion (deck of cards size).
Good Source	Provides 10–19% Daily Value for the nutrient stated (fiber, calcium, vitamin A or K).
Excellent Source	Provides at least 20% Daily Value for the nutrient stated (fiber, calcium, vitamin A or C).

5. When there is a strong relationship between a nutrient or food component and health, a *health claim* may appear on the label. The product must meet certain criteria for such claims to be allowed.

Recommended Dietary Allowances (RDAs) for Adults
(10th edition, National Research Council)

The Recommended Dietary Allowance for each vitamin and mineral listed below is the average level of intake that will meet the nutritional needs of most healthy people. For some nutrients, there is not enough scientific information to establish an RDA, so only an "estimated safe and adequate" daily dietary intake is listed. Because even fewer conclusions are possible regarding sodium and potassium intakes, only an estimate of the minimum requirements for good health are stated.

Vitamins and Minerals

The following lists indicate those foods that are especially high in specific vitamins and minerals. A balanced diet should provide sufficient amounts of these nutrients.

VITAMINS

Vitamin A
Beneficial to vision, reproduction, growth, immune function; mucous membranes, bone, skin, hair, and teeth need Vitamin A for proper de-

	Adult Male (19–24 years)	Adult Male (25–50 years)	Adult Male (51+ years)	Adult Female (19–24 years)	Adult Female (25–50 years)	Adult Female (51+ years)
VITAMINS						
Vitamin A	1,000 RE*	1,000 RE	1,000 RE	800 RE	800 RE	800 RE
B-Complex						
B1 (thiamin)	1.5 mg	1.5 mg	1.2 mg	1.1 mg	1.1 mg	1.0 mg
B2 (riboflavin)	1.7 mg	1.7 mg	1.4 mg	1.3 mg	1.3 mg	1.2 mg
B3 (niacin)	19 mg	19 mg	15 mg	15 mg	15 mg	13 mg
B6 (pyridoxine)	2.0 mg	2.0 mg	2.0 mg	1.6 mcg	1.6 mcg	1.6 mcg
B12 (cobalamin)	2.0 mcg	2.0 mcg	2.0 mcg	2.0 mcg	2.0 mcg	2.0 mcg
Folate	200 mcg	200 mcg	200 mcg	180 mcg	180 mcg	180 mcg
Vitamin C	60 mg	60 mg	60 mg	60 mg	60 mg	60 mg
Vitamin D	10 mcg	5 mcg	5 mcg	10 mcg	5 mcg	5 mcg
Vitamin E	10 mg	10 mg	10 mg	8 mg	8 mg	8 mg
Vitamin K	70 mcg	80 mcg	80 mcg	60 mcg	65 mcg	65 mcg
MINERALS						
Calcium	1200 mg	800 mg	800 mg	1200 mg	800 mg	800 mg
Iodine	150 mcg	150 mcg	150 mcg	150 mcg	150 mcg	150 mcg
Iron	10 mg	10 mg	10 mg	15 mg	15 mg	10 mg
Magnesium	350 mg	350 mg	350 mg	280 mg	280 mg	280 mg
Phosphorus	1200 mg	800 mg	800 mg	1200 mg	800 mg	800 mg
Selenium	70 mcg	70 mcg	70 mcg	55 mcg	55 mcg	55 mcg
Zinc	15 mg	15 mg	15 mg	12 mg	12 mg	12 mg

*Retinal Equivalents

Estimated safe and adequate daily dietary intakes for adults of various vitamins and minerals

Biotin	30–100 mcg	Fluoride	1.5–4.0 mg
Chromium	50–200 mcg	Pantothenic Acid	4.0–7.0 mg
Copper	1.5–3.0 mg		

Estimated minimum requirements for healthy adults

Potassium	2000 mg	Sodium	500 mg

velopment and maintenance. Beta-carotene, a precursor of Vitamin A found in some fruits and vegetables, may be protective against heart disease due to its antioxidant properties.

Cereals (fortified)
Eggs
Fruits (especially apricots, cantaloupe, mangoes, peaches)
Organ meats (liver and kidney)
Margarine

Milk
Vegetables (broccoli, carrots, pumpkin, spinach, sweet potato,
    red pepper, winter squash)

B-complex
*These vitamins are all necessary for the proper metabolism of carbo-
hydrate, protein, and fat. They are also needed for normal functioning
of the nervous, muscular, and cardiovascular systems and for maintenance of skin, nails, and hair.*

Thiamine (B1)
Beef (lean)
Breads and cereals (whole grain, enriched or fortified)
Eggs
Fish
Nuts
Organ meats
Pork and ham
Poultry
Rice
Sunflower seeds
Wheat germ

Riboflavin (B2)
Cereals (enriched or fortified)
Cheese (especially cheddar and cottage)
Eggs
Fish
Liver
Milk
Nuts
Pork
Poultry
Yogurt
Vegetables (asparagus and spinach)
Wheat germ

Niacin (B3)
Beans
Beef
Cereals (enriched or fortified)
Corn

Fish (especially bluefish, halibut, salmon, swordfish, tuna)
Lamb
Liver
Nuts and peanut butter
Peas
Poultry
Sunflower seeds
Wheat bran

Pyridoxine (B6)

Bananas
Beans (especially soy and white)
Beef
Cereals (fortified)
Eggs
Fish (especially bluefish, halibut, mackerel, snapper, salmon)
Nuts (especially peanut butter, filberts, walnuts)
Organ meats
Pork and ham
Poultry
Prunes
Sunflower seeds

Cobalamin (B12)

Found only in animal foods.
Beef
Cheese
Eggs
Fish (especially bluefish, mackerel, salmon, snapper, trout, tuna)
Lamb
Milk
Organ meats
Pork
Shellfish (especially clams, crab, lobster, oysters, mussels)
Yogurt

Pantothenic Acid

Chicken
Cottage cheese
Fish (especially herring, mackerel, salmon, sole, trout, tuna)
Lamb

Liver
Lobster
Oatmeal
Vegetables (especially broccoli, cauliflower, corn, sweet
    potatoes)
Wheat germ

Folate
*Necessary for synthesis of red and white blood cells and for function-
ing of the nervous and gastrointestinal systems.*

Beans (garbanzo, lima, pinto)
Cereals (fortified)
Eggs
Nuts
Orange juice
Vegetables (especially asparagus, mustard and turnip greens,
    romaine lettuce, spinach)

Biotin
*Beneficial to circulation and integrity of hair and skin. Needed for me-
tabolism of foods.*

Cereals
Eggs
Fish
Nuts
Oats and oatmeal
Organ meats
Wheat bran

Vitamin C
*Needed for healing of wounds and healthy bones, skin, and teeth.
Helps in manufacturing red blood cells. Controversial as to whether it
helps prevent or speed recovery from the common cold.*

Cereals (fortified only)
Fruits and fruit juices (especially cantaloupe, grapefruit,
    honeydew, kiwi, mango, orange, pineapple, raspberries,
    strawberries, tangerine)
Potatoes (sweet and white, baked)
Vegetables (especially broccoli, Brussels sprouts, cabbage,
    cauliflower, kale, green or red pepper, mustard greens,
    rutabaga, spinach, tomatoes and tomato juice, turnip
    greens)

Note: Cook vegetables in a minimum amount of water or steam them to retain as much vitamin C as possible.

Vitamin D

Necessary for proper bone development and maintenance. Helps with absorption of calcium and phosphorus. The body can manufacture Vitamin D from exposure to at least 15 minutes of sunlight per day.

Eggs
Fish (especially bluefish, flounder, herring, perch, salmon, sardines, sole, trout, tuna)
Liver
Margarine
Milk (fortified)
Pork (hot dogs, salami, sausage)
Pudding and custard
Shellfish (especially oysters, shrimp)

Vitamin E

Primary function is to act as an antioxidant that protects body tissues from damage. May be protective against heart disease, but studies are not conclusive.

Fish (especially mackerel and salmon)
Granola cereal
Hummus
Margarine
Mayonnaise
Nuts and peanut butter
Olives
Salad dressing
Shellfish (oysters, shrimp)
Vegetables (green leafy varieties primarily: Brussels sprouts, cabbage, collard greens, dandelion greens, kale, sweet potatoes)
Vegetable oils
Wheat germ

Vitamin K

Plays an important role in blood clotting.

Green leafy vegetables (especially broccoli, cabbage, kale, lettuce, turnip greens, spinach)
Green tea

MINERALS

Calcium

Major function is development and maintenance of bones and teeth. Also beneficial to blood clotting, heart, and nervous system. Primarily derived from dairy products, but some other foods below are notable sources.

> Broccoli
> Cereal (if fortified with calcium)
> Cheese
> Fish (those with bone consumed such as canned salmon, sardines)
> Ice cream and ice milk
> Milk
> Orange juice (if fortified with calcium)
> Pudding and custard
> Yogurt (including frozen yogurt)

Chromium

Essential for the metabolism of foods, especially carbohydrates, and for blood sugar control.

> Bran
> Liver
> Meats
> Seafood (especially oysters)
> Whole grain breads and cereals

Copper

Necessary for many metabolic processes.

> Bran cereal
> Liver
> Mushrooms
> Nuts and seeds
> Shellfish (especially clams, crab, lobster, oysters)

Fluoride

Important for development and maintenance of bones and teeth.

> Foods and beverages prepared with fluoridated water
> Tea
> Water (if fluoridated)

Iodine
Essential for production of thyroid hormones.
- Fish (saltwater varieties)
- Salt (iodized)
- Seafood
- Water

Iron
Beneficial to red blood cell production and the immune system.
- Beans
- Beef (lean)
- Cereals (bran, whole grain or fortified)
- Dried fruit (apricots, prunes, raisins)
- Liver
- Molasses (blackstrap)
- Nuts and seeds
- Sardines
- Shellfish (clams, oysters)
- Tofu

Magnesium
Needed for normal cardiac and neurologic functioning.
- Bread (if whole grain)
- Cereals (bran and whole grain)
- Halibut
- Molasses (blackstrap)
- Nuts and seeds
- Potato
- Spinach
- Tofu

Phosphorus
Essential for development and maintenance of teeth and bones.
- Beans
- Cereals (bran or whole grain)
- Cheese
- Eggs
- Fish and shellfish (especially clams, crab, flounder, lobster, scallops, shrimp)
- Meats (including beef, lamb, liver, pork)
- Milk

Nuts and seeds
Poultry

Potassium

An electrolyte integral to fluid balance of the muscular and nervous systems.

Beans
Cereals (bran)
Fish and shellfish (especially bluefish, clams, flounder, salmon, swordfish)
Fruits (especially bananas, cantaloupes, grapefruit juice, honeydew, nectarines, oranges, raisins)
Meats and poultry
Milk and milk products
Nuts and peanut butter
Potatoes
Vegetables (especially beet greens, broccoli, Brussels sprouts, carrots, chard, collard greens, corn, peas, pumpkin, spinach, sweet potatoes, tomatoes and tomato products, winter squash)

Note: In order to preserve potassium content, steam vegetables and do not boil potatoes.

Selenium

Necessary for metabolism; has antioxidant properties.

Beef
Fish and shellfish
Nuts and seeds
Organ meats

Zinc

Beneficial to the metabolism of protein, carbohydrates, and fat and to taste buds.

Beef (lean)
Cereals (bran, whole grain or fortified)
Cheese (Swiss)
Lamb
Liver
Milk and milk products
Pork
Poultry (especially dark meat)
Shellfish (especially clams, crab, oysters)

Nutritional Supplements

Each year, consumers spend billions of dollars on nutritional supplements. Many people are looking for increased energy and vitality, while others have heard that large doses of a certain vitamin, mineral, or food supplement will prevent or cure a particular disease. The truth is that a person who is healthy and who eats a balanced diet should be getting the amount of vitamins and minerals needed according to the Recommended Dietary Allowances (RDAs). Obtaining vitamins and minerals from food is best because other nutrients, such as complex carbohydrates, fiber, and protein, are also obtained. A vitamin or mineral supplement is appropriate under some circumstances:

- When you do not eat the recommended number of servings from one or more food groups in the Food Guide Pyramid for an extended period of time whether due to a hectic lifestyle, food preferences, or personal beliefs. Many women do not consume enough servings from the dairy group to get the required amount of calcium. Strict vegetarians are at risk for several deficiencies, including vitamins B12, D, and riboflavin as well as calcium and iron.

- Pregnant or lactating women need more iron, folate, and calcium. Prenatal supplements are recommended by many physicians.

- Diets that contain fewer than 1,200 calories a day, even when very well planned, will, most likely, lack one or more nutrients.

If a nutritional supplement is taken, read labels and find one that provides no more than 100% of the RDA for vitamins and minerals. Doses of vitamins and minerals far beyond the RDA can be dangerous, especially for the fat soluble vitamins A, D, E, and K. The saying "If some is good, more is better" does not apply to nutrition. There is no difference in the body's utilization of natural versus synthetic vitamins and minerals. The natural versions are likely to be an unwarranted added expense.

What of claims that high doses of a particular nutrient or nutritional supplement can ward off or treat diseases? Claims are made that vitamin C helps the common cold, that vitamin E prevents heart disease and cancer, and that fish oils, garlic, or niacin lower cholesterol levels. While there have been new and promising research findings about many nutrients and supplements, do not confuse these with a recommendation to start taking all sorts of pills, potions, and powders.

Often, the dosages required are so high that, without the supervision of your physician, more harm than good can be done. Always ask your doctor before taking any nutritional supplements.

7-DAY MENU PLAN: Basic Healthy Diet

The following menu plan conforms to the Dietary Guidelines for Americans and consists of approximately 2,200 calories. Foods generally thought of as "bad" (because they are somewhat high in fat, sodium, or sugar) can be incorporated into a diet if these choices are exercised in moderation and balanced by more nutritious selections. Depending upon food preferences and individual calorie needs, adjust the menus accordingly by using the Composition of Foods table (pages 62–225) as a guide. To reduce the calories in this plan, consider eliminating the desserts and sweets; reducing the amount of added fats or using reduced fat versions of salad dressings, mayonnaise, or margarine; and eating smaller portions of most foods. For those who need to eat more calories, there is room for larger serving sizes, but try to avoid too many from the top of the Food Guide Pyramid, such as sweets and added fats.

Note: All margarine is tub form from corn oil. Oils used in food preparation are preferably canola, olive, or corn. The portion sizes listed for meat, fish, poultry, rice, stuffing, hot cereal, and hot vegetables are based on weight or cup measurement *after* cooking. Beverages such as plain coffee or tea, water, and sugar-free beverages have negligible nutritional value and can be used freely. The meal plan can be adjusted to include other beverages such as soft drinks or juice.

SUNDAY
Breakfast
> ¼ cup orange juice
> 3 pancakes, grilled using about 1 tsp. canola oil and topped with
> > 1 tsp. tub margarine and 3 Tbsp. maple syrup
> 2 strips bacon
> 1 cup 1% fat milk

Lunch
> Hamburger on a bun:
> > 3 ounces extra-lean ground beef, broiled
> > Hamburger bun, preferably whole wheat

1 Tbsp. catsup
Lettuce and tomato
20 oven-baked steak fries with 1 Tbsp. catsup

Dinner
Chicken stir-fry using 2 tsp. canola oil:
4 ounces skinless chicken breast
1 cup mixed vegetables such as pea pods, carrots, bean
sprouts, mushrooms, broccoli, water chestnuts
Soy sauce, preferably reduced-sodium version
1 cup brown rice
1 cup fresh fruit salad

Snacks and Treats
1 small ice cream cone

MONDAY
Breakfast
½ grapefruit
1 bagel, preferably wheat or whole grain
2 Tbsp. cream cheese

Lunch
Tuna salad sandwich:
½ cup tuna with small amount of mayonnaise
2 slices pumpernickel bread
Lettuce and tomato
1 cup low-fat fruit yogurt
1 pear

Dinner
5 ounces roast pork, trimmed
2 medium boiled potatoes
2 spears broccoli
2 tsp. tub margarine
½ cup unsweetened applesauce

Snacks and Treats
6 low-fat crackers, preferably unsalted tops
2 Tbsp. peanut butter
1 cup 1% fat milk

TUESDAY
Breakfast
> ¾ cup orange juice
> 1 cup bran flakes cereal
> 1 cup 1% fat milk
> ½ banana

Lunch
> Turkey sandwich:
>> 3 ounces turkey breast
>> 2 slices whole wheat bread
>> Lettuce and tomato
>> 2 tsp. mayonnaise
> 1 large apple

Dinner
> Tossed salad with 1 Tbsp. vinaigrette dressing
> Spaghetti with meatballs:
>> 2 cups cooked spaghetti noodles
>> 2 medium meatballs (about 4 ounces lean or extra-lean
>>   ground beef)
>> ½ cup marinara sauce
> 2 slices Italian bread with 2 tsp. olive oil or tub margarine

Snacks and Treats
> 4 gingersnap cookies
> 1 cup 1% fat milk

WEDNESDAY
Breakfast
> ¾ cup orange juice
> 1 English muffin, preferably whole wheat
> 1 Tbsp. jam
> 1 scrambled egg, using about 1 tsp. tub margarine and 1% fat
>   milk

Lunch
> Chef's salad:
>> Mixed greens, tomato, and 1 ounce each ham, turkey, and
>>   cheese

2 Tbsp. Italian dressing
4 sesame bread sticks
20 grapes

Dinner

4 ounces roasted or grilled chicken, no skin
1 baked potato with 1 tsp. tub margarine and 1 Tbsp. sour cream
½ cup stuffing, prepared from mix with tub margarine
1 cup peas and carrots
1 whole wheat dinner roll
1 tsp. tub margarine
4 pineapple slices in own juice

Snacks and Treats

1 cup 1% fat milk
4 fig bar cookies

THURSDAY
Breakfast

1 cup cooked oatmeal with 1 tsp. tub margarine and 1 Tbsp.
   honey
1 cup fresh fruit salad
1 cup 1% fat milk

Lunch

Ham sandwich:
   2 ounces lean deli ham, preferably low salt
   2 slices rye bread
   2 tsp. mustard
½ cup coleslaw
1 ounce potato chips
1 cup apple cranberry juice

Dinner

2 cups beef and vegetable stew (1 cup vegetables, 5 ounces
   trimmed stew meat, and 1 tsp. canola oil per serving)
1 cup yolk-free egg noodles
1 medium-sized sourdough roll
1 tsp. tub margarine

Snacks and Treats
1 cup ice milk

FRIDAY
Breakfast
½ grapefruit
1 bran muffin
1 Tbsp. jam and 2 tsp. tub margarine
1 cup 1% fat milk

Lunch
1 bowl lentil soup
8 wheat crackers with 1 oz. reduced-fat cheese spread
1 large apple

Dinner
6 ounces baked or broiled flounder
1 cup wild rice
1 cup stir-fried green beans with almonds (1 cup green beans, 1
Tbsp. chopped blanched almonds, and 1 tsp. olive oil)
2 slices whole grain bread with 2 tsp. tub margarine

Snacks and Treats
1 small piece homemade blueberry pie (⅛th of a 9-inch pie),
using vegetable shortening in crust

SATURDAY
Breakfast
¾ cup orange juice
Mushroom, onion, and pepper omelet, prepared with 1 tsp.
canola oil (2 eggs: to reduce cholesterol intake, replace one of
the eggs with 2 egg whites)
2 slices wheat toast
2 tsp. tub margarine
½ cantaloupe
Coffee or tea

Lunch
1 cup chili with beans (using extra-lean ground beef)
1 cup rice, preferably brown rice
1 small piece cornbread

Dinner

Tossed salad with 1 Tbsp. vinaigrette dressing
3 slices cheese pizza from large pie

Snacks and Treats

2 plums

General recommendations for a sensible weight-loss diet resemble the guidelines for a healthy, balanced diet. They involve eating a variety of foods but reducing the overall number of calories consumed. The easiest way to accomplish this is by eating fewer foods that are high in fat or sugar content and by limiting alcohol, which can be a substantial source of empty calories. Also, concentrate on eating more fiber, including whole grains, fruits, and vegetables. Most of these foods are naturally low in fat and calorie content. In addition, increasing fiber will add bulk to the diet and will help to provide a feeling of fullness. Choose more skinless poultry and fish because they usually contain less fat (especially saturated fat) and calories than most cuts of beef, pork, or lamb. Dairy products should be low- or non-fat to save on calories and fat.

Eat a variety of the proper foods according to the Food Guide Pyramid in moderation, including at least:

6 servings a day from the bread and cereal group

2–4 servings of vegetables;

3 servings from the fruit group;

2 servings from the meat and meat alternatives group; and

2 servings (low- or non-fat) of milk and milk products.

Fats such as butter, margarine, mayonnaise, and oil should be used very sparingly. Try to bake, broil, grill, poach, or steam foods instead of frying them. To sauté items without extra fat and calories, use a non-stick skillet and vegetable cooking spray. To add flavor and variety to foods, use a splash of lemon or lime juice, garlic, spices, and herbal vinegar instead of calorie- and fat-laden gravies and sauces. For dessert, try fresh fruit, sugar-free gelatin, graham crackers, and low-fat frozen yogurt. But remember that low-fat or fat-free frozen desserts and baked goods can be a substantial source of calories that should be counted into your total calorie allotment. Beverages may also contribute calories to your diet. Drink as many calorie-free liquids as possible.

Budget calories by eating a little less at some meals to allow for extra calories at parties and special occasions. However, do not skip meals. Be sure to make exercise part of your weight-loss regime. Exercising for at least half an hour a day will increase the number of calories burned. Refer to the Calories Burned with Exercise chart on page

29 for an idea of how many calories are burned per hour with various types of activities.

Adopt healthy eating habits that will enable you to lose weight and to keep it off as well. A weight loss of 1–2 pounds a week is considered reasonable and safe. Adult males tend to lose excess weight faster than adult females. If you experience the so-called dieter's plateau—a stretch of time during which there is very little or no weight loss despite adherence to an eating and exercise plan—be patient. This slowdown happens to almost everyone and is usually temporary. Adhere to a program of healthy eating and exercise and your goal will be reached. Consult the chart on page 227 to determine ideal weight.

One question often asked is, "How many calories do I need to eat per day to lose weight?" This depends upon a person's age, body size, and level of physical activity. To lose one pound of weight per week, a person needs to trim 500 calories a day (3,500 calories a week) from the amount currently being eaten or 1,000 calories a day (7,000 a week) to lose 2 pounds a week. To understand better where the calories are coming from, keep track of what is eaten for several typical days, using the Food Diary (pages 228–229). Then, begin to alter food selections, preparation methods, and/or portion sizes to deduct the necessary calories. To define more closely calorie needs for weight loss, use the worksheet on page 28. A diet consisting of fewer than 1,200 calories a day is not recommended unless it is supervised by a health care provider.

Two restricted-calorie diets with 7-day menu plans for each appear on the following pages. Generally, the 1,200-calorie plan is appropriate for individuals who are less active or when a faster weight loss (2 pounds a week) is desired, while the 1,800-calorie diet is more suitable for slower weight loss (one pound a week) or for more active persons.

Calculating Your Calorie Quota

The following is a method for estimating roughly the calorie needs for healthy, nonpregnant adults, ages 18–50 years. Older individuals should further reduce calories by 10% to 20%.

A. Refer to the chart on page 227 and determine a realistic ideal weight in the range shown for your height.

Generally, the higher weights in the range apply to men, who usually have more muscle and bone mass than most women. The lower weights in the range more often apply to women.

IDEAL WEIGHT _____ pounds

B. Classify yourself by lifestyle.

_____ Less Active   Little or no regular exercise, desk job

_____ Active   Moderate level of regular exercise, active at work

_____ Very Active   Strenuous regular exercise, manual labor at work

C. Determine your energy need by multiplying your Ideal Weight by your activity level:

Less Active = 13   Active = 15   Very Active = 17

_____ × _____ = _____ Calories a day
(This is the level of calories that will be needed for weight maintenance once your goal weight is achieved.)

D. Subtract calories for weight loss.

_____ − 500 = _____ Calories a day to lose 1 pound a week
(Calories from
section C)

_____ − 1000 = _____ Calories a day to lose 2 pounds a week
(Calories from
section C)

Note: The lowest recommended calorie intake is 1200 calories a day, even if it would slow down the rate of weight loss. Diets of fewer than 1200 calories a day tend to be nutritionally inadequate.

DAILY CALORIE GOAL = _____

Calories Burned with Exercise

Weight loss is best accomplished by a sensible reduced-calorie diet and exercise. It takes a deficit of 3,500 calories, accomplished by eating less and/or exercising more, to lose one pound. The amount of calories burned depends upon several factors including body size, body composition, age, gender, and the intensity of the exercise performed. The chart below gives a general idea of the amount of calories burned per hour during various activities. Most women should use the values at the lower end of the range, while the upper range is usually appropriate for men.

Activity	Calories Burned per Hour
Aerobics, light	345–445
Aerobics, moderate	425–550
Aerobics, step, moderate	625–825
Baseball	275–350
Basketball, easy game	400–500
Biking/cycling, 6 m.p.h.	250–325
Cleaning	175–250
Dancing	325–425
Gardening, moderate	275–375
Golf, walking with bag	400–500
Hiking, moderate	275–375
Jogging/running, 10 min. mile	575–750
Jogging/running, 6 min. mile	900–1200
Laundry	175–250
Mowing, self-propelled mower	200–275
Nordic track, moderate	525–700
Racquetball, moderate	550–725
Shopping	200–275
Shoveling snow	375–475
Skiing, downhill	375–475
Stairmaster, 60 steps/min.	400–500
Swimming, moderate	325–450
Tennis, moderate	375–475
Walking, 20 min. mile	175–250
Walking, 15 min. mile	225–300

Values derived from the Food Processor Plus Nutrition Analysis Systems, ESHA Research, Salem, Oregon.
Reference subjects: 40-year-old woman, 5'5" tall, 140 pounds; 40-year-old man, 5'11" tall, 180 pounds. You may burn more calories if you are younger, taller, or heavier than reference subjects and fewer calories if you are shorter, older, or lighter than reference subjects.

7-DAY MENU PLAN: 1,200 Calories

Note: All margarine is tub form from corn oil. Oils used in food preparation are preferably canola, olive, or corn. The portion sizes listed for meat, fish, poultry, rice, stuffing, pasta, hot cereal, and hot vegetables are based upon weight or cup measurement *after* cooking. Beverages such as plain coffee or tea, water, or sugar-free soft drinks have a negligible nutritional value and can be used freely. Be sure to count the calories of other fluids such as regular soda, punch, or juice.

Diets of 1,200 calories or less tend to be low in calcium and fiber if not carefully planned. Use high-fiber bread and grain products and calcium-fortified foods (some cereals, juices, and breads) whenever possible.

SUNDAY
Breakfast
> ½ cup orange juice
> 2 pancakes, grilled using about 1 tsp. canola oil and topped with
>   2 Tbsp. low-calorie maple syrup
> 1 cup 1% fat milk

Lunch
> Hamburger on a bun:
>   2 ounces extra-lean ground beef, broiled
>   Hamburger bun, preferably whole wheat
>   1 Tbsp. catsup
>   Lettuce and tomato
> ½ cup fresh fruit salad

Dinner
> Chicken stir-fry using 2 tsp. canola oil:
>   3 ounces skinless chicken breast
>   1 cup mixed vegetables such as pea pods, carrots, bean
>   sprouts, mushrooms, broccoli, water chestnuts
>   Soy sauce, preferably reduced-sodium version
> ½ cup brown rice
> ½ cup low-fat frozen yogurt

MONDAY
Breakfast
> ½ grapefruit
> 1 bagel, preferably wheat or whole grain
> 2 Tbsp. low-fat cream cheese

Lunch
> Tuna salad sandwich:
>   2 oz. tuna in water with 1 Tbsp. low-fat mayonnaise

2 slices low-calorie oat bran bread
Lettuce and tomato
½ cup low-fat fruit yogurt with artificial sweetener
1 small pear

Dinner

3 ounces roast pork, trimmed
1 medium boiled potato
3 spears broccoli
1 tsp. tub margarine
½ cup unsweetened applesauce
1 cup 1% fat milk

TUESDAY
Breakfast

½ cup orange juice
½ cup bran flakes cereal
1 cup 1% fat milk
½ banana

Lunch

Turkey sandwich:
  2 ounces turkey breast
  2 slices low-calorie whole wheat bread
  Lettuce and tomato
  1 tsp. mayonnaise
1 apple
1 cup 1% fat milk

Dinner

Tossed salad with 1 Tbsp. low-calorie Italian dressing
Spaghetti with meatballs:
  1 cup cooked spaghetti
  2 small meatballs (about 3 ounces lean or extra-lean ground beef)
  ¼ cup marinara sauce

WEDNESDAY
Breakfast

½ cup orange juice
1 English muffin, preferably whole wheat

1 Tbsp. sugar-free jam
1 scrambled egg, using about 1 tsp. tub margarine and 1% fat milk (as needed)

Lunch

Chef's salad
    Mixed greens, tomato, and 1 ounce each turkey and low fat cheese
    2 Tbsp. low calorie Italian dressing
2 sesame breadsticks
15 grapes
1 cup 1% fat milk

Dinner

3 ounces grilled chicken
1 small baked potato with 1 tsp. tub margarine and 2 Tbsp. low-fat sour cream
1 cup cooked peas and carrots
4 pineapple slices in own juice

THURSDAY
Breakfast

1 cup cooked oatmeal with 1 tsp. tub margarine and 1 Tbsp. honey
½ cup fresh fruit salad
1 cup 1% fat milk

Lunch

Ham sandwich:
    2 ounces lean deli ham, preferably low salt
    2 slices low calorie rye bread
    2 tsp. mustard
Carrot and celery sticks
1 orange

Dinner

1½ cups beef and vegetable stew (1 cup vegetables, 3 ounces trimmed stew meat, and about 1 tsp. canola oil per serving)
½ cup yolk-free egg noodles
½ cup low-fat frozen yogurt

FRIDAY
Breakfast
½ grapefruit
1 small bran muffin
2 tsp. tub margarine
1 cup 1% fat milk

Lunch
1 cup lentil soup
6 wheat crackers
1 apple

Dinner
5 ounces baked or broiled flounder
½ cup wild rice
1 cup stir-fried green beans with almonds (1 cup green beans,
     1 Tbsp. chopped blanched almonds, and 1 tsp. olive oil)
½ cup sugar-free gelatin with 2 unsweetened canned peach
     halves

SATURDAY
Breakfast
½ cup orange juice
Mushroom, onion, and pepper omelet, prepared using nonstick
     spray (1 egg)
1 slice wheat toast
1 tsp. tub margarine
¼ cantaloupe
1 cup 1% fat milk

Lunch
1 cup chili with beans (using extra-lean ground beef)
2 plums

Dinner
Tossed salad with 1 Tbsp. low-calorie dressing
2 slices cheese pizza from large pie

7-DAY MENU PLAN: 1,800 Calories

Note: Optional: Plain coffee or tea, water, dietetic beverages. Be sure to count the calories of other beverages such as regular soft drinks, punch, or juice. All margarine is from corn oil. Fats allotted for food preparation are included in the meal plan. Otherwise, use nonstick cooking spray. The portion sizes listed for meat, poultry, fish, rice, stuffing, pasta, hot cereal, and hot vegetables are based upon weight or cup measurements *after* cooking.

SUNDAY
Breakfast
⅓ cup orange juice
2 pancakes, grilled using about 1 tsp. canola oil and topped with
    1 tsp. tub margarine and 2 Tbsp. maple syrup
1 cup 1% fat milk

Lunch
Hamburger on a bun:
    3 ounces extra-lean ground beef, broiled
    Hamburger bun, preferably whole wheat
    1 Tbsp. catsup
    Lettuce and tomato
10 oven-baked steak fries with 1 Tbsp. catsup

Dinner
Chicken stir-fry using 2 tsp. canola oil:
    4 ounces skinless chicken breast
    1 cup mixed vegetables such as pea pods, carrots, bean
        sprouts, mushrooms, broccoli, water chestnuts
    Soy sauce, preferably reduced-sodium version
1 cup brown rice
1 cup fresh fruit salad

Snacks and Treats
1 small low-fat frozen yogurt cone

MONDAY
Breakfast
½ grapefruit
1 bagel, preferably wheat or whole grain
1 Tbsp. cream cheese

Lunch

Tuna salad sandwich:
- ½ cup tuna with small amount of mayonnaise
- 2 slices pumpernickel bread
- Lettuce and tomato
1 cup low-fat fruit yogurt
1 pear

Dinner

4 ounces roast pork, trimmed
1 medium boiled potato
2 spears broccoli
1 tsp. tub margarine
½ cup unsweetened applesauce

Snacks and Treats

6 low-fat crackers, preferably unsalted tops
1 Tbsp. peanut butter
1 cup 1% fat milk

TUESDAY

Breakfast

½ cup orange juice
1 cup bran flakes cereal
1 cup 1% fat milk
½ banana

Lunch

Turkey sandwich:
- 2 ounces turkey breast
- 2 slices whole wheat bread
- Lettuce and tomato
- 1 tsp. mayonnaise
1 cup 1% fat milk

Dinner

Tossed salad with 1 Tbsp. vinaigrette dressing
Spaghetti with meatballs:
- 2 cups cooked spaghetti noodles
- 2 medium meatballs (about 4 ounces lean or extra-lean ground beef)

½ cup marinara sauce
1 slice Italian bread with 1 tsp. olive oil or tub margarine

Snacks and Treats
1 apple

WEDNESDAY
Breakfast
½ cup orange juice
1 English muffin, preferably whole wheat
1 Tbsp. jam
1 scrambled egg, using tub margarine and 1% fat milk

Lunch
Chef's salad:
Mixed greens, tomato, and 1 ounce each ham, turkey, and
cheese
2 Tbsp. Italian dressing
3 sesame breadsticks
20 grapes

Dinner
4 ounces roasted or grilled chicken, no skin
1 medium-sized baked potato with 1 tsp. tub margarine
1 cup cooked peas and carrots
1 whole wheat dinner roll
1 tsp. tub margarine
1 cup 1% fat milk

Snacks and Treats
4 pineapple slices in own juice

THURSDAY
Breakfast
1 cup cooked oatmeal with 1 tsp. tub margarine and 1 Tbsp.
honey
1 cup fresh fruit salad
1 cup 1% fat milk

Lunch
> Ham sandwich:
>> 2 ounces lean deli ham, preferably low salt
>> 2 slices rye bread
>> 2 tsp. mustard
> 1 ounce potato chips
> 1 cup apple cranberry juice

Dinner
> 2 cups beef and vegetable stew (1 cup vegetables, 5 ounces
>> trimmed stew meat, and 1 tsp. canola oil per serving)
> 1 cup yolk-free egg noodles
> 1 small slice sourdough bread
> 1 tsp. tub margarine

Snacks and Treats
> ½ cup low-fat frozen yogurt

FRIDAY
Breakfast
> ½ grapefruit
> 1 bran muffin
> 2 tsp. tub margarine
> 1 cup 1% fat milk

Lunch
> 1 bowl lentil soup
> 6 wheat crackers
> 1 apple

Dinner
> 6 ounces baked or broiled flounder
> 1 cup wild rice
> 1 cup stir-fried green beans with almonds (1 cup green beans,
>> 1 Tbsp. chopped blanched almonds, and 1 tsp. olive oil)
> 1 slice whole grain bread with 1 tsp. tub margarine

Snacks and Treats
> ½ cup gelatin with 3 peach halves

SATURDAY

Breakfast

½ cup orange juice

Mushroom, onion, and pepper omelet, prepared with 1 tsp.
canola oil (2 eggs: To reduce dietary cholesterol intake,
replace one of the eggs with 2 egg whites)

1 slice wheat toast

1 tsp. tub margarine

1/4 cantaloupe

Lunch

1 cup chili with beans (using extra-lean ground beef and 1 tsp.
olive or canola oil)

½ cup rice, preferably brown rice

Dinner

Tossed salad with 1 Tbsp. vinaigrette dressing

3 slices cheese pizza from large pie

Snacks and Treats

2 plums

SPECIAL DIETS

Low-Sodium Diet

Sodium is a mineral that plays a major role in regulating fluid balance in the body. An excessive sodium intake can increase the risk of developing high blood pressure and can further increase blood pressure in individuals with known hypertension. A low-sodium diet is recommended for individuals with certain kidney, heart, and liver disorders and when some medications may interfere with normal fluid balance. Even for healthy individuals, moderation in sodium intake is recommended.

The National Research Council recommends an average daily intake of no more than 2,400 mg of sodium a day for healthy people. Sodium can be further restricted in the treatment of particular medical conditions such as uncontrolled hypertension, congestive heart failure, and liver and kidney diseases associated with fluid retention. The minimum amount of sodium needed for health is 500 mg a day, or the amount in ¼ teaspoon of table salt. Most Americans take in far more sodium than is necessary or desirable.

The major source of sodium in the typical American diet is table salt (sodium chloride) that is used in food preparation, at the table, and in the manufacture of processed, prepared, and convenience food items. The food industry has developed many low- and reduced-sodium products that are widely available. Refer to the section Reading Food Labels (page 8) for more information. While sodium does occur naturally in most foods, the amount is usually small. In general, diets are lowest in sodium when very little processed, prepared, and convenience foods are used and when whole grains, fresh fruits, vegetables, and meat, fish, and poultry (all prepared without salt) are emphasized.

GENERAL GUIDELINES:

1. Omit or reduce the use of table salt, salt-based spices, and high-sodium condiments. Use more herbs, spices, lemon juice, or herbal vinegars for flavor. Only use salt substitutes with permission of your physician as they contain more potassium than is desirable for some people.

2. Buy as many fresh foods as possible, and limit the use of processed, prepared, and convenience foods.

3. When canned, frozen, or packaged foods are purchased, check the labels to identify the sodium content *per serving* of that item.

Avoid purchasing items with claims such as "reduced sodium" or "light in sodium" and, instead, identify the milligrams of sodium per serving. Foods that contain more than 480 mg of sodium per serving should be used less frequently.

4. Refer to the list of foods below, which are typically significant sources of sodium. Foods not appearing on the list contain some natural sodium but not in high quantities.

Foods to Limit or Avoid

Bread, Cereal, Rice, and Pasta

Cake mixes (especially angel food and chocolate; check labels)
Cereals (some dry and instant hot varieties; check labels)
Cornbread, commercially prepared or from mix
Mixes for biscuits and pancakes, especially buttermilk-type
Macaroni, rice, and stuffing mixes
Prepared frozen macaroni and cheese, pancakes and waffles
Salted crackers
Salted snack foods (cheese curls, popcorn, potato chips, pretzels, snack mixes, tortilla chips)
Seasoned bread crumbs and croutons

Fruits

Maraschino cherries
Some dried fruits (check labels)

Vegetables

Brine-cured (sauerkraut, olives) and marinated (artichoke hearts) vegetables
Canned, unless without added salt
Frozen with sauce
Pickled (pickled beets, pickles, three bean salad)
Potato mixes, including instant potato flakes
Spaghetti sauce and canned tomato products

Milk, Yogurt, and Cheese

Buttermilk
Cheeses (including Parmesan; reduced- or low-sodium types are available; check labels)
Cheese sauces and spreads
Malted milk and malted milk drink mixes
Pudding, instant mix

Meat, Poultry, Fish, Eggs, and Nuts
Bacon
Beans (baked beans, canned—unless well rinsed, pork and beans)
Canned items (including anchovies, chicken, chili, chipped beef, chow mein, corned beef and corned beef hash, ham and deviled ham, meat spreads, salmon, sardines, seafood, stews, tuna)
Fast foods
Frankfurters (except low-sodium types)
Frozen TV dinners, entrees, fish fillets, fried or breaded chicken (most)
Kielbasa
Luncheon meats (most, except "low-sodium" varieties)
Nuts, if salted
Pizza
Sausage
Smoked fish, meats, and poultry

Fats, Oils, and Sweets
Gravy mixes
Salad dressing (most)
Salt pork

Miscellaneous
Bacon bits
Barbecue sauce
Catsup (unless low sodium; use regular types very sparingly)
Meat tenderizers
Monosodium glutamate (MSG)
Prepared mustard (use very sparingly)
Relish
Salsa
Salt, including "lite" types and salt-based spices such as garlic salt, onion salt, and seasoned salt; read labels on spice mixes as there may be hidden sodium (some lemon-pepper spices)
Sauce mix packages and bottled sauces
Steak sauce
Soups and broth (canned, condensed, cubes, dehydrated; some reduced- or low-sodium varieties acceptable)
Soy sauce, including "lite" types
Tartar sauce
Teriyaki sauce

Heart Healthy Eating

Most Americans eat too much fat, saturated fat, and cholesterol, which are major factors in the development of heart disease. High blood cholesterol levels can often be treated by a diet containing lesser amounts of these nutrients.

Not all types of blood cholesterol are undesirable. For example, a type of cholesterol called low density lipoprotein, or "LDL," can promote atherosclerosis or plaque buildup in the arteries that supply blood to the heart. High density lipoprotein, or "HDL," another type of cholesterol, is protective against heart disease. A diet that is too high in saturated fat and cholesterol can increase LDL cholesterol levels and lower HDL cholesterol levels. All adults should have their blood cholesterol level checked—ask your physician.

GUIDELINES FOR IMPLEMENTATION

1. The calories in your diet should be appropriate for achieving and maintaining your ideal weight (see Suggested Weights for Adults, p. 227, and Calculating Your Calorie Quota, p. 27). Being too fat, especially if you are apple-shaped, can increase LDL and lower HDL cholesterol.

2. Obtain 30% or less of your calories from total fat. To calculate fat requirements, first determine overall calorie needs. By multiplying calorie needs by 0.30, the daily diet of fat calories can be determined. Then divide fat calories by 9, the number of calories per gram of fat. This will result in the recommended fat gram allowance per day.

   EXAMPLE: 1,800 calories $\times$ 0.30 = 600 fat calories
   600 fat calories $\div$ 9 = 67 grams of fat

3. About 10% of daily calories or less should be from saturated fat. This is the type of fat found in animal products as well as solid vegetable fats and tropical oils.

   EXAMPLE: 1,800 calories $\times$ 0.10 = 180 saturated fat calories
   180 saturated fat calories $\div$ 9 = 20 grams of saturated fat

Replace saturated fats with unsaturated sources. Polyunsaturated fats include safflower, soybean, sunflower, and corn oil, and margarine made with these oils. Avoid using hydrogenated sources such as sticks of margarine, vegetable shortening, and products prepared with hydrogenated vegetable oil as the first type of fat in the list of ingredients. Hydrogenation appears to increase the amount of another undesirable fat called *trans* fat. Monounsaturated fats are olive, peanut, and canola oils. Overall, monounsaturated fats are preferable but should still be used as part of the total fat allowance.

4. Limit dietary cholesterol, which is found only in animal foods, to 300 mg a day. Accomplish this by choosing up to 6 oz. a day of lean sources from the meat and meat alternatives group and by limiting eggs, shellfish, and organ meats.

5. Take in adequate amounts of fiber, particularly soluble fiber as found in beans, lentils, fresh fruits, oats, and barley.

6. If following the above guidelines does not optimize your blood cholesterol levels, reduce dietary cholesterol intake to 200 mg a day and saturated fat to 7% or less of daily calories. At this point, seek the assistance of a registered dietitian.

7. Individuals with a high level of triglycerides (a type of blood fat) should avoid alcoholic beverages and limit high sugar foods in addition to the above.

Many experts feel that further reducing total fat intake to as low as 10% of daily calories is appropriate. This may be effective for some types of cholesterol elevations but not all. Very low-fat, high-carbohydrate diets may worsen HDL cholesterol and elevate triglycerides in some people. Be sure to check with your physician before making drastic dietary changes.

MEAL PLANNING TIPS

1. Many foods from the bread, rice, cereal, and pasta group are very low in fat content (0–1 gram of fat per serving). Focus on choices highest in fiber. Limit the use of snack foods and bakery goods, as they contain a considerable amount of fat. Be sure to count the fats used in preparing these foods. As a spread on top of breads, try jam. Reduced-fat soft margarine and sour cream can be used on top of vegetables or potatoes. Fat-free baked goods are acceptable, but be careful as they often have a high calorie count.

2. Fruits and vegetables by nature contain virtually no fat, saturated fat, or cholesterol. Enhance vegetables by using lemon juice, herbal vinegar, or reduced-fat and fat-free salad dressing. If vegetables are stir-fried, use only a small amount of an acceptable oil or non-stick cooking spray.

3. Dairy products should be low fat. Look for 1% fat milk, low-fat yogurt, and cheese with fewer than 3 grams of fat per ounce.

4. Choose fish and skinless chicken more often than red meat. When using red meat, buy lean cuts such as extra-lean ground beef, top round, sirloin steak, flank steak, eye round, center, loin or tenderloin pork, leg of lamb, or shoulder lamb chops. Shellfish can be used occasionally, but limit the frequency due to its relatively high cholesterol content. Many luncheon meats, hot dogs, and sausage products are available with an acceptable fat content (read labels to find products that contain fewer than 3 grams of fat per ounce or 10 grams of fat per 3-ounce portion).

   Limit egg yolks to about 3 per week, including what has been used in food preparation. Use egg substitutes or replace one whole egg with two egg whites. Use organ meats infrequently.

   Trim off all visible fat from these foods before preparing them, and use methods such as baking, broiling, roasting, poaching, or grilling as they do not require extra added fat. Above all, keep portion sizes to no more than 6 ounces daily (about the size of 2 decks of cards).

   Some meat alternatives, such as dry beans and peas, contain no fat, saturated fat, or cholesterol. Try to incorporate some "vegetarian" entrees into your diet, such as meatless chili or lentil soup.

5. All added fats should be used in moderation, including unsaturated sources. Regular tub margarine, mayonnaise, and vegetable oils contain about 5 grams of fat per teaspoon, so using them liberally may bankrupt your fat budget quickly. Reduced fat or "diet" margarine and mayonnaise contain about 5 grams of fat per 1 tablespoon portion. Use more herbs and spices to enhance food flavors. Added fats can often be reduced in quantity or even eliminated entirely.

6. Use alcohol in moderation. Certain alcoholic beverages, such as red wine, may be beneficial for preventing heart disease in some people since it appears to raise protective HDL cholesterol. Remember that alcohol can be a source of excess calories and can in-

teract with many medications. People with high triglyceride levels may make this condition worse by drinking alcohol.

High-Fiber Diet

Fiber, also known as roughage, is the undigestible portion of plant foods. Fiber helps with proper functioning of the intestinal tract as it speeds the elimination of waste products. Because a high-fiber diet alleviates constipation, it is a likely preventive against colon cancer as there is less exposure of cancer causing agents to the intestinal tract. Other intestinal ailments such as diverticulosis, asymptomatic diverticulitis, hemorrhoids, and irritable bowel can be prevented and/or treated with a high-fiber diet.

Individuals with diabetes may also benefit from a high-fiber diet since it may improve blood sugar control. Soluble fiber, a type of fiber found in oats, legumes, barley, and some fruits, may help reduce blood cholesterol levels. On a weight-loss diet, fiber may improve success as high-fiber foods (especially vegetables and fruits) tend to be low in calorie content, take a long time to chew, and are quite filling. Most authorities recommend at least 25 grams of fiber daily (some say up to 40 grams a day), but most Americans eat far less. Milk and dairy products, meat, fish and shellfish, poultry, eggs, and fats have an insignificant amount of fiber. Fiber is not broken down as a result of cooking foods.

GUIDELINES FOR IMPLEMENTATION

1. Increase the fiber in the diet slowly to prevent abdominal bloating, gas, and flatulence.

2. Soak beans or lentils overnight in water and rinse well to reduce their gassiness and lessen cooking time.

3. Wash fruits and vegetables well. Try not to remove the skin or peel whenever possible as this usually reduces the fiber content. Choose fresh or even canned fruits over juice.

4. Fiber should be obtained from a variety of whole grains, breads and cereals, fruits, and vegetables. Take a fiber supplement only if recommended by a physician.

5. Fruits and vegetables with small seeds (berries, figs, tomatoes) as well as poppy or sesame seeds should be used with caution by individuals with a history of diverticular disease.

6. Drink an adequate amount of fluids; otherwise, a high-fiber diet may be constipating. Aim for 6–8 glasses a day.

7. Read food labels to compare the grams of fiber per serving among similar food items, choosing those with the highest fiber content. Use refined grains less frequently.

8. Refer to the list below for more information on the fiber content of various foods.

Fiber Content of Various Foods

6+ grams of fiber per serving

Bread, Cereal, Rice, Pasta, and Meat Alternatives

Beans, cooked (½ cup): baked, kidney, navy, pinto, refried, white

Bean soups (1 cup)

Black-eyed peas, cooked (½ cup)

Cold cereals (⅓ cup): 100% Bran, All Bran, Bran Buds, Fiber One

Hummus (¼ cup)

Vegetables

Artichokes (1 globe)

Baby lima beans, cooked (½ cup)

Fruits

Blackberries (1 cup)

Prunes, stewed (½ cup)

4.1–6.0 grams of fiber per serving

Bread, Cereal, Rice, Pasta, and Meat Alternatives

Beans, cooked (½ cup): black, garbanzo, lima

Cold cereals (¾ cup): Bran Chex, Bran Flakes, Corn Bran, Mueslix, Raisin Bran

Grains, cooked (½ cup): bulgur wheat, barley

Lentils, cooked (½ cup)

Oatmeal, cooked (1 cup)

Oat bran, dry (⅓ cup)

Pumpkin seeds, roasted (¼ cup)

Split pea soup (1 cup)

Fruits

Guava (1)

Mango (1)

Pear (1)
Raspberries (1 cup)
Strawberries (1 cup)

Vegetables
Acorn squash, cooked (½ cup)
Brussels sprouts, cooked (½ cup)
Fordhook lima beans, cooked (½ cup)

3.1–4.0 grams of fiber per serving
Bread, Cereal, Rice, Pasta, and Meat Alternatives
Bran or oat bran muffin (1)
Cold cereals: Grapenuts (⅓ cup), granola (½ cup), Shredded Wheat (¾ cup)
Nuts (¼ cup): almonds, mixed nuts
Popcorn (3 cups) and popcorn cakes (2)
Wheat germ (¼ cup)
Whole wheat English muffin (1) or pita bread (1)

Fruits
Blueberries (1 cup)
Figs, fresh or dried (2)
Orange (1)
Papaya (1 cup)

Vegetables
Butternut and winter squash, baked, mashed (½ cup)
Corn on the cob (1 ear)
Kale, raw (1 cup)
Peas, cooked (½ cup)
Sweet potato (1)

2.0–3.0 grams of fiber per serving
Bread, Cereal, Rice, Pasta, and Meat Alternatives
Boston brown bread (1 slice)
Cold cereals (¾ cup): Oat Flakes, Wheat Chex, Wheaties
Crackers: Rye Crisp or Flatbread (2), Stoned Wheat (6), Triscuits (6), Wheat Thins (12)
Grains (½ cup), buckwheat groats (kasha), couscous
Instant oatmeal
Nuts: cashews, peanuts (¼ cup), chunky peanut butter (2 Tbsp.)

Sunflower seeds, dry roasted (¼ cup)
Whole wheat and mixed grain breads (1 slice) (check labels as fiber
    content varies)
Whole wheat pasta (½ cup)

Fruits
Apple (1)
Banana (1)
Coconut, dried, flaked (¼ cup)
Dates (4)
Kiwi (1)
Nectarine (1)
Pears, canned (½ cup)
Raisins (¼ cup)

Vegetables
Broccoli, cooked (½ cup)
Carrots, cooked (½ cup)
Collard greens, cooked (½ cup)
Corn, canned or frozen (½ cup)
Parsnips, cooked (½ cup)
Pea pods/snow peas (½ cup)
Potato, including skin (1 med.)
Pumpkin, cooked (½ cup)
Sauerkraut (½ cup)
Spaghetti sauce (½ cup)
Spaghetti squash (½ cup)
Spinach, cooked (½ cup)
Yellow or wax beans, cooked (½ cup)

Foods with less than 2.0 grams of fiber per serving are listed under the Low-Fiber Diet. These foods can also be included in your diet, but unless eaten in great quantity, they will not provide adequate fiber.

Food Ideas:
● Add cooked beans to soups, stews, and casseroles or on top of salads.

● Substitute whole wheat and rye flour in place of all-purpose flour, brown rice for white rice, and spinach or whole wheat pasta for standard pasta.

- Incorporate bran or rolled oats in such main dishes as meatloaf or casseroles.

- Sprinkle a high-fiber cereal on top of your favorite breakfast cereal, mix it into yogurt, or use as topping on frozen desserts.

- Use fruits as snacks and desert and even try a main dish that incorporates fruit, such as pineapple and chicken.

- Add vegetables to main dishes, casseroles, soups, and stews.

Diabetic Diet

A healthy diet for people with diabetes is very similar to the Dietary Guidelines for Americans. Foods high in fiber and naturally low in fat should be emphasized, such as whole grains, fresh fruits, and vegetables. Dairy products should be low fat, while meat and meat alternative selections should focus on lean sources with about 6 ounces total per day. Added fats and sugars should be used sparingly. Calories should be consumed to attain a healthy weight. Protein should comprise about 10–20% daily calories, fats about 30% daily calories. The remaining calories should come from carbohydrate (about 50% daily calories). The exact breakdown of calories can vary, depending upon blood glucose levels and the presence of other medical conditions such as a high blood cholesterol or triglyceride level.

For nearly a century, people with diabetes were told to avoid simple carbohydrates (such as table sugar, maple syrup, and corn syrup) because they dramatically increase blood glucose levels. Instead, starches or complex carbohydrates (such as bread, rice, potatoes, cereals, and pastas) were encouraged. Recent guidelines do not strictly prohibit the use of simple carbohydrates because there is insufficient proof that they raise blood sugar any more than starches. Instead, as with everyone, sugar in all its forms should be used in moderation. Fructose, a natural sugar found in fruit, fruit juice concentrates, and honey, can also be used in moderation. There is probably no benefit to blood sugar from using fructose instead of sucrose or table sugar. It is now recommended that the diabetic diet focus on the total amount of carbohydrate (about 50% daily calories) as opposed to the form of carbohydrate obtained. If sugars are used, they should be counted as part of the carbohydrate allowed each day and not just an extra item added into the diet. Because foods high in sugar are often high in calories and provide few vitamins and minerals, they should not be overused.

Individuals with insulin-dependent diabetes (type I) need to pay close attention to consistency in meal and snack composition, size, and times to keep blood sugar as near normal levels as possible. Additional planning is needed to avoid and treat hypoglycemia, especially when one is sick or has exercised more than usual.

Those with non-insulin-dependent diabetes (type II) often need to focus on reaching a healthy weight, getting more exercise, and, like all Americans, eating less fat, saturated fat, cholesterol, sodium, and sugar. A weight loss of 10–20 pounds can improve blood glucose levels for many people.

In summary, there is no longer any one "correct" diabetic diet. In addition to the Dietary Guidelines for Americans, other strategies for a healthy diabetic diet include using the Exchange Lists for Meal Planning by the American Diabetes Association and the American Dietetic Association and counting carbohydrate grams. A registered dietitian (R.D.) can help develop a meal plan that is best suited for an individual's needs and includes the foods the individual enjoys eating, even some sugary foods on occasion.

For more information, contact the American Diabetes Association at 1-800-232-3472. The Nutrition Consumer Hotline at the National Center for Nutrition and Dietetics, 1-800-366-1655, can help you locate a registered dietitian in your area.

Vegetarian Diet

A vegetarian is someone who excludes one or more types of animal products. There are several types of vegetarians. A *lacto-ovo-vegetarian* excludes meat, fish, poultry, and seafood but does include milk, milk products, and eggs. A *lacto-vegetarian* will further exclude eggs, while a *vegan* only eats plant foods. *Semi-vegetarians* usually consume some type of fish or poultry but do not eat red meats.

Since vegetarian diets focus on foods at the base in the Food Guide Pyramid, they have the potential to be lower in fat, saturated fat, and cholesterol and higher in fiber content than the typical American diet. Except for a vegan diet, the other vegetarian diets can be nutritionally adequate if wisely chosen. Vegans need to supplement vitamin B12 (found only in animal foods) or consistently include foods fortified with this nutrient, such as many soybean products. Calcium, zinc, iron, vitamin D, and riboflavin may also be low in this very restrictive diet.

Diets that include eggs and/or milk and milk products will provide high quality protein in which all essential amino acids should be present. Plant foods contain protein, but usually of lower quality because one or more essential amino acids is lacking or low.

GUIDELINES FOR IMPLEMENTATION

1. Generally speaking, it is recommended that foods from the bread, rice, and pasta group be combined with either vegetables, legumes, or nuts or seeds (meat alternatives) to ensure that the amino acids naturally low in this group are obtained from another. However, it is no longer considered critical to have certain combinations or "complementary" proteins in the same meal, but rather to focus on a variety of foods from each group over the entire day. Meal suggestions using plant foods include:

Sautéed vegetables with brown rice	Couscous with vegetables
Pasta and beans	Hummus on pita bread
Lentil soup with peanut butter and crackers	Vegetable salad topped with nuts/seeds
Vegetarian chili with cornbread	Stir-fried tofu with vegetables over rice

2. Pay careful attention to the nutrients that may be lacking in a diet, based upon which foods are excluded, and use nutritional supplements as appropriate.

3. Adapt the food groups below for meal planning based upon individual preferences:

Foods Allowed

Bread, Cereal, Rice, and Pasta
Whole grain bread, cereals, rice, and pasta
Baked goods prepared without animal fat

Fruits and Vegetables
All, including texturized vegetable protein products

Meat Alternatives
Eggs (for lacto-ovo-vegetarians)
Nuts, peanut butter, seeds
Legumes (cooked dry beans, peas, lentils, peanuts)
Tofu (soybean curd)

Milk and Milk Products
All (for lacto- and lacto-ovo-vegetarians)

Fats and Sugars
Vegetable oil, vegetable shortening, margarine
Sugar, jam, jelly, honey, corn syrup

Lactose-Restricted Diet

Many people are not able to fully digest lactose, the type of sugar found in milk and milk products, due to a deficiency of an enzyme called lactase. Symptoms of lactose intolerance include abdominal bloating, stomach cramps, and diarrhea. Consult a doctor if a lactose intolerance is suspected.

GUIDELINES FOR IMPLEMENTATION

1. Tailor the diet to meet a personal level of tolerance for lactose. Some people can tolerate small amounts of lactose, particularly from fermented milk products such as aged cheeses.

2. Unless adequate calcium is consistently obtained from non-dairy sources, talk with a doctor about taking a calcium supplement.

3. Reduced-lactose dairy products such as milk or cheese are available, but they are usually not completely lactose-free. Lactase enzyme has been added to these products to "predigest" most of the lactose. Use these products if they are tolerated to help create a diet more nutritionally balanced and adequate in calcium. Ask a doctor about the use of over-the-counter lactase enzyme preparations.

4. Always read labels to identify hidden sources of lactose from food processing. Key words to look for include milk, milk solids, non-fat dry milk, milk powder, whey, curd, and lactose. Avoid foods with these ingredients. Lactic acid, lactalbumin, and lactate do not contain lactose or milk and can safely be used.

5. Refer to the list below of foods to avoid or strictly limit.

Foods to Avoid:
Bread, Cereal, Rice, and Pasta
Any product prepared with milk or milk solids; check label
Some cold and instant hot cereals

Products prepared with butter or milk-containing margarine
Rice and pasta mixes with dehydrated cheese, cream, or milk solids
Most baking mixes, including pancake mix

Vegetables
Creamed vegetables
Vegetables or potatoes prepared with butter or milk-containing
  margarine
Frozen vegetables and potatoes if processed with lactose
Instant potato flakes and mixes with dehydrated cheese or cream
  sauce

Fruits
Canned or frozen if processed with lactose

Meat, Poultry, Fish, Dry Beans and Peas, Eggs, and Nuts
Eggs prepared with milk, cheese, butter, or milk-containing
  margarine
Cold cuts and hot dogs with milk solids
Creamed or many breaded meat, fish, or poultry items

Milk and Milk Products
Cheese
Cocoa mixes
Ice cream, ice milk, frozen yogurt, sherbet
Custard, mousse, and pudding
Milk, buttermilk, chocolate milk, evaporated milk, malted milk,
  sweetened condensed milk (some people may be able to use milk
  treated with lactase)
Yogurt

Fats and Sugars
Butter
Cream and cream sauces
Gravy if containing butter, milk-containing margarine, cream, or milk
  solids
Margarine containing milk
Salad dressings containing milk or milk products
Sour cream
Some candies: butterscotch, caramels, chocolate, toffee

Miscellaneous
Soups prepared with milk or cream
Canned soup or dry mixes containing milk or nonfat milk solids

Foods Allowed
(Always check labels)

Bread, Cereal, Rice, and Pasta
Products prepared without butter, milk-containing margarine, milk, or
    milk solids (usually includes hard rolls, French and Italian
    breads, soda crackers, angel food cake)
Cooked plain cereal
Pasta, rice

Vegetables
Plain fresh, canned, or frozen to which no lactose has been added

Fruits
Plain fresh, canned, or frozen to which no lactose has been added

Meat, Poultry, Fish, Dry Beans and Peas, Eggs, and Nuts
Kosher cold cuts and hot dogs
Plain beef, chicken, lamb, organ meats, pork, poultry, veal
Eggs, poached, boiled, or prepared with acceptable ingredients
Peanut butter, nuts, seeds, and cooked dry beans and peas

Milk and Milk Products
Some people may tolerate a small amount of milk products, including
    lactase-treated milk and cheese

Fats and Sugars
Milk-free margarine
Many non-dairy creamers
Oils
Salad dressing without milk or milk solids
Vegetable shortening
Fruit ice, sorbet, gelatin
Sugar, jam, jelly, honey, corn syrup, most hard candy

Dietary Guidelines for Gout

The occurrence of gout is associated with a diet that is excessive in purine content. Purines are normally converted into uric acid, which is then eliminated in the urine. In people prone to gout, uric acid levels are often high due to an increased rate of formation of uric acid and to a diminished rate of excretion. When uric acid builds up in the bloodstream, crystals are formed that can then deposit in the joints. These deposits cause a painful inflammation and can also be responsible for uric acid kidney stones. It is recommended that individuals with gout avoid an excessive purine intake so that less uric acid is produced.

Much of the purines in the typical American diet are obtained from animal proteins such as meat, poultry, fish, and shellfish. It is therefore recommended that serving sizes of these foods be kept to about 5 to 7 ounces daily. The difference in calories can be made up with foods high in carbohydrate, such as breads, grains, fruits, and vegetables. A high carbohydrate diet actually helps increase the excretion of uric acid.

Asparagus, mushrooms, and spinach contain a moderate amount of purine. Cooked dried beans and peas (kidney beans, white beans, chickpeas, black-eyed peas, etc.) and lentils also contain a substantial amount of purine. They can, however, be used *in place of* meat, fish, or poultry as an alternative source of protein.

The foods highest in purine content to be avoided are:

Anchovies

Bouillon, broth, consomme, and meat-based soups

Goose

Gravy

Herring

Mackerel

Meat-based extracts (used in gravies, sauces, soups, processed foods)

Mincemeat

Mussels

Organ meats, including brains, heart, kidney, liver, pancreas (sweetbreads)

Partridge

Roe (fish eggs)

Scallops

Yeast

Other nutritional factors such as consuming excessive fat or alcohol, being overweight, and not drinking enough fluid are known to negatively affect uric acid levels. In addition to the above, it is suggested that one attain or maintain an ideal body weight and lose any excess weight slowly (rapid weight loss may increase uric acid levels); keep fat intake to no more than 30% of daily calories; drink alcohol in moderation; and drink 6–8 glasses of water daily.

Diet for Reactive Hypoglycemia

Reactive hypoglycemia is a condition resulting in a low blood sugar level about 1–5 hours after a meal and then resolving spontaneously. This is different from the hypoglycemia associated with insulin or other medications for diabetes. Characteristics of reactive hypoglycemia include weakness, feeling faint, anxiety, and hunger. Diagnosis of reactive hypoglycemia can be made only through laboratory testing by a physician.

There is much disagreement about what type of diet is best for reactive hypoglycemia. Often, the appropriate regimen can only be determined on a trial and error basis. If a doctor has diagnosed reactive hypoglycemia, try the following suggestions as a start:

1. Attain and maintain your ideal body weight by eating the appropriate number of calories and engaging in regular physical activity.

2. Eat three meals and two to three snacks a day. Be consistent about meal times and do not skip meals or snacks. Meals and snacks should encompass a variety of foods so that a mixture of protein, fat, and carbohydrate is obtained.

3. There is some evidence that foods high in sugar (thus high in total carbohydrate) should be strictly limited. This includes items such as cake, candy, cookies, danish, doughnuts, honey, maple syrup, pie, sweetened cereal, canned fruits and juices, most frozen

desserts, regular soda, pudding, and gelatin. These foods are probably best tolerated as part of a meal, as opposed to a snack.

4. The carbohydrates chosen should be complex sources such as whole grain breads and cereals, beans or lentils, rice, pasta, or potatoes. Focus on the choices that are highest in fiber content, particularly soluble fiber as found in fresh fruits, beans or lentils, barley, and oats.

5. People vary in the amount of total carbohydrate tolerated. Adjust your diet according to what alleviates your symptoms.

6. It you drink alcohol, do so in moderation. Alcohol is best tolerated as part of a meal.

High-Calcium Diet

The 10th edition of the Recommended Dietary Allowances suggests 800 mg of calcium a day for adults ages 25–50. For adults ages 18–24 years and for pregnant or lactating women, 1,200 mg of calcium a day is recommended. Many scientists believe that this amount of calcium may not be sufficient to prevent osteoporosis, a condition in which bone loss occurs, increasing the risk of bone fractures. In addition to inadequate calcium intake, other controllable lifestyle risk factors for osteoporosis include inadequate exercise, cigarette smoking, lack of other nutrients such as vitamin D, and excessive intake of alcohol, sodium, and protein.

At a minimum, be sure to meet the RDA for calcium, preferably from food sources. It appears that taking in even more calcium than the RDA may be beneficial. If osteoporosis is diagnosed, ask a doctor how much calcium is needed, as it is often much higher than the RDAs listed above.

Below is a list of foods that are rich in calcium. The portion size listed provides about 300 mg of calcium. To meet the RDA, 3–4 servings a day from this list are needed. To keep calories, fat, and cholesterol intakes in balance, use low-fat dairy products.

Food	Portion Size for 300 mg calcium
Bread, calcium fortified	2 slices
Broccoli	4 cups
Cheese, natural	1.5 oz.
Cheese, processed	2 oz.

Cottage cheese	2 cups
Ice cream	2 cups
Juice, calcium fortified	1 cup
Milk	1 cup
Pudding	1 cup
Ricotta cheese	½ cup
Salmon, canned with bone	5 oz. (1 cup)
Sardines	7
Total cereal	1½ cups
Turnip greens	1½ cups
Yogurt, carton or frozen	1 cup

Read labels to evaluate foods for their calcium content. A food that is a good source of calcium will provide at least 10% daily value for calcium. If a diet cannot be altered to get adequate calcium, discuss the use of calcium supplements with a physician.

Low-Fiber Diet

Physicians sometimes recommend a low-fiber (also called fiber-restricted) diet (about 10 grams of fiber a day) for individuals with intestinal problems. During the acute phases of Crohn's disease, ulcerative colitis, and diverticulitis, or after intestinal surgery, a low-fiber diet decreases the amount of waste products that need to be eliminated so that the intestinal tract is not aggravated or irritated. In some cases, a low-residue diet is advised, which further limits the use of dairy foods and any meats with tough connective tissues.

Note that cooking, mashing, or puréeing foods does not change their fiber content. However, cooked (including canned) fruits and vegetables may cause less gas and are often more easily tolerated than raw fruits or vegetables.

GUIDELINES FOR IMPLEMENTATION

1. Whenever possible, use refined grains such as all-purpose flour and white rice.

2. Remove the skin or peel from fruits and vegetables and the tough membranes from meat.

3. Avoid breads and crackers with nuts, bran, poppy, rye, or sesame seeds.

4. Avoid fruit pies and other desserts that may have nuts, coconut, raisins, or small seeds (blueberry pie, pecan pie).

5. Milk and milk products, meat, poultry, fish and shellfish, and fats do not contain fiber. If "residue" should be limited per doctor's orders, use only tender meats and milk products in moderation.

Foods to Limit or Avoid

Refer to the High-Fiber Diet (page 45) for foods higher in fiber content (more than 2.0 grams of fiber per serving) that should be avoided or used in extreme moderation.

Foods Allowed

1.0–2.0 grams of fiber per serving
Bread, Cereal, Rice, Pasta, and Meat Alternatives
Apple pie (1 small slice)
Bagel, plain or egg (1)
Breads (1 slice): French, Italian, white; some rye, oat, pumpernickel, and wheat breads (read labels carefully)
Bread stuffing (½ cup)
Brown rice, cooked (½ cup)
Corn bread (1 piece), corn muffin (1), corn tortilla (1), or tortilla chips (1 oz.)
Dry cereal (¾ cup) (check labels)
English muffin (1)
Hot cereal (1 cup): Cream of Rice, Cream of Wheat
Pasta (½ cup)
Peanut butter, smooth (2 Tbsp.)
Rye bread (1 slice)
Spinach pasta, cooked (½ cup)
Tortilla, flour (1)

Fruits
Applesauce (½ cup)
Apricots, canned halves (½ cup), fresh (2)
Cantaloupe (1 cup)
Fruit cocktail, canned (½ cup)
Grapefruit (½)
Peaches, canned (½ cup), fresh (1 med.)
Pineapple slices, canned (½ cup)
Plums, canned (½ cup), fresh (2 med.)

Vegetables

Asparagus (½ cup)

Beet greens (½ cup)

Beets, cooked (½ cup)

Cabbage, cooked (½ cup)*

Cauliflower, cooked (½ cup)*

Celery, raw (2 stalks)

Egg noodles, cooked (½ cup)

Eggplant, cooked (½ cup; remove seeds)

Green or red pepper, cooked (½ cup)*

Leeks, cooked (½ cup)

Mushrooms, cooked (½ cup)

Mustard greens, raw (1 cup)

Okra, cooked (½ cup; remove seeds)

Onions, cooked (½ cup)*

Potatoes, baked, no skin (1 med.), hash browns (½ cup), mashed
(½ cup)

Spinach, raw (1 cup)

String beans (½ cup)

Tomatoes, whole (1), canned (½ cup; remove seeds)

Turnips, cooked (½ cup)

Water chestnuts (½ cup)

Zucchini, cooked (½ cup; remove seeds)

*May be too gaseous for some people

Less than 1.0 gram of fiber per serving
Bread, Cereal, Rice, Pasta, and Meat Alternatives

Blueberry muffin, from mix (1)

Biscuits

Breads (1 slice): egg, French, Italian, pita (white), sourdough, Vienna,
white

Crackers: butter-type (6), Graham (3), Melba toast (6), Saltines (1)

Dry cereal (¼ cup)

Rice cake

White rice

Fruits

Cherries (12)

Fruit juices without pulp (½ cup)

Grapes (12)

Mandarin oranges, canned (½ cup)

Tangerine (1)
Watermelon (1 cup)

Vegetables
Bamboo shoots, canned (½ cup)
Cucumber, peeled (½; remove seeds)
Lettuce, raw (1 cup)
Radishes (6)

COMPOSITION OF FOODS

The table that follows presents more than 1,000 commonly eaten foods—in the forms that consumers find when shopping or dining out. The table gives the typical serving size for each food and then shows the amounts of the vital elements: calories, fat (total and saturated), cholesterol, sodium, carbohydrate (including fiber), and protein. To calculate calories from fat, multiply fat grams by 9. To convert both carbohydrate and protein grams into calories, multiply by 4.

The foods are listed in alphabetical order. When there are several varieties of a general type of food, such as baby foods, beverages, or frozen meals, they are listed under the general heading.

Use this table to get a general idea of the nutritional value of the foods you normally eat. Check food labels for the exact amount of a particular nutrient, as brands can vary significantly. Refer to Reading Food Labels (p. 8) for further details.

Food	Amount	Calories	Total Fat (gm)	Saturated Fat (gm)
A				
Almonds, dried, unblanched	1.0 oz.	168	14.9	1.4
Apple, fresh, with skin	1 med.	82	.5	.1
Apple butter	1 Tbsp.	33	.1	0
Apple juice canned or bottled	1 c.	118	.3	.1
frozen concentrate, unsweetened, diluted per directions	1 c.	115	.2	trace
Applesauce sweetened	½ c.	97	.2	trace
unsweetened	½ c.	52	.1	trace
Apricot nectar	1 c.	140	.2	trace
Apricots canned, heavy syrup, with skin	1 c.	213	.2	trace
dried, uncooked	¼ c.	77	.2	trace

*A dash (–) in a column indicates no reliable data even though component may be present in a measurable amount.

Cholesterol (mg)	Sodium (mg)	Carbohydrates (gm)		Protein (gm)
		Total	Fiber	
0	3.1	5.8	.8	5.7
0	0	21.2	1.1	.3
0	0	8.5	.1	trace
0	8	29.3	.5	.2
0	17	28.0	0	.3
0	4	25.5	.6	.2
0	2	13.8	.6	.2
0	8	36.0	.5	.9
0	10	55.1	1.0	1.4
0	3	20.1	1.0	1.2

Food	Amount	Calories	Total Fat (gm)	Saturated Fat (gm)
Apricots *(cont'd)* fresh	3	51	.4	trace
Artichokes cooked	½ c.	42 (varies fresh to stored)	.1	trace
raw	1 lg. head	76 (varies fresh to stored)	.3	.1
Asparagus canned	1 c.	48	1.8	.3
fresh, spears, cooked	4 spears	14	.2	trace
frozen cuts and tips, cooked	4 spears	17	.2	.1
Avocado California	1	305	29.9	4.5
Florida	1	339	81.5	5.5

Cholesterol (mg)	Sodium (mg)	Carbohydrates (gm)		Protein (gm)
		Total	Fiber	
0	1	11.8	.6	1.5
0	79	9.3	1.1	2.9
0	152	16.9	1.9	5.3
0	880	6.3	0	5.2
0	6	2.5	.5	1.5
0	2	2.9	.5	1.8
0	21	11.9	3.6	3.6
0	15.2	27.0	6.4	4.8

Food	Amount	Calories	Total Fat (gm)	Saturated Fat (gm)

B

Food	Amount	Calories	Total Fat (gm)	Saturated Fat (gm)
Baby foods–Cereals and cereal products, precooked, dry Barley	1 oz.	106	1	0
High-protein	1 oz.	105	1.7	0
Mixed	1 oz.	110	1.3	0
Oatmeal	1 oz.	115	2.3	0
Rice	1 oz.	114	1.4	0
Teething biscuit	1 oz.	114	1.2	0
Baby foods–Desserts, dinners, meats, poultry, eggs, commercially prepared in jars, bottles, or cans **_Desserts_** Custard pudding (all flavors)	3.5 oz.	85	2.0	0
Fruit pudding	3.5 oz.	59	0	0

Cholesterol (mg)	Sodium (mg)	Carbohydrates (gm)		Protein (gm)
		Total	Fiber	
0	14	21.8	.3	3.2
0	14	13.5	.7	10.4
0	11	21.3	.3	3.5
0	10	20.1	.3	3.9
0	9	22.5	.2	2.1
0	105	22.2	.1	3.1
0	28	16.1	0	1.6
0	14	16.0	.2	.3

Food	Amount	Calories	Total Fat (gm)	Saturated Fat (gm)
Dinners (cereal, vegetable, meat mixtures, 2–4% protein) Beef noodle dinner	3.5 oz.	53	1.7	0
Chicken noodle dinner	3.5 oz.	52	1.5	0
Macaroni, tomatoes, meat, and cereal	3.5 oz.	55	1.1	0
Split peas, vegetables, and ham	3.5 oz.	71	1.3	0
Meats, poultry, and eggs Beef, junior	3.5 oz.	106	4.9	2.6
Beef, strained	3.5 oz.	107	5.4	2.6
Beef, with vegetables	3.5 oz.	75	4.2	0
Chicken	3.5 oz.	130	7.9	2.0
Chicken, with vegetables	3.5 oz.	78	3.6	0
Lamb, junior	3.5 oz.	112	5.2	2.6

Cholesterol (mg)	Sodium (mg)	Carbohydrates (gm)		Protein (gm)
		Total	Fiber	
0	29	7.0	.3	2.3
0	16	7.5	.3	2.1
0	17	8.8	.4	2.2
0	14	11.3	.3	3.3
0	66	0	0	14.5
0	81	0	0	13.6
0	36	4.2	.3	5.7
0	47	.1	0	13.7
0	27	5.9	.2	6.2
0	73	0	0	15.2

Food	Amount	Calories	Total Fat (gm)	Saturated Fat (gm)
Baby foods, *Meats (cont'd)* Lamb, strained	3.5 oz.	103	4.7	2.3
Liver, strained	3.5 oz.	101	3.8	1.4
Pork, strained	3.5 oz.	124	7.1	2.4
Turkey, with vegetables	3.5 oz.	87	4.8	0
Veal, strained	3.5 oz.	101	4.8	2.3
Baby foods–Fruits and fruit products, with or without thickening Applesauce	3.5 oz.	41	.2	0
Applesauce and apricots	3.5 oz.	45	.2	0
Bananas, strained, with tapioca or cornstarch, added ascorbic acid	3.5 oz.	57	.1	0
Bananas and pineapple, with tapioca or cornstarch	3.5 oz.	68	.1	0

Cholesterol (mg)	Sodium (mg)	Carbohydrates (gm)		Protein (gm)
		Total	Fiber	
0	62	.1	0	14.1
183	74	1.4	0	14.3
0	42	0	0	14.0
0	30	6.0	.1	5.6
0	64	0	.1	13.5
0	2	10.9	.5	.2
0	3	11.6	.7	.2
0	9	15.3	.2	.4
0	8	18.4	0	.2

Food	Amount	Calories	Total Fat (gm)	Saturated Fat (gm)
Baby foods—Fruits *(cont'd)* Fruit dessert with tapioca (apricot, pineapple, and/or orange)	3.5 oz.	60	0	0
Peaches	3.5 oz.	71	.2	0
Pears	3.5 oz.	41	.2	0
Pears and pineapple	3.5 oz.	41	.1	0
Plums with tapioca, strained	3.5 oz.	71	0	0
Prunes with tapioca	3.5 oz.	70	.1	0
Baby foods— Vegetables Beans, green	3.5 oz.	25	.1	0
Beets, strained	3.5 oz.	34	.1	0
Carrots	3.5 oz.	27	.1	0
Mixed vegetables (including vegetable soup)	3.5 oz.	41	.5	0

Cholesterol (mg)	Sodium (mg)	Carbohydrates (gm)		Protein (gm)
		Total	Fiber	
0	8	16.3	.3	.3
0	6	18.9	.7	.5
0	2	10.8	0	.3
0	4	10.9	.3	.3
0	6	19.7	0	.1
0	5	18.5	.3	.6
0	2	5.9	1.0	1.3
0	83	7.7	.8	1.3
0	37	6.0	.8	.8
0	13	8.0	.4	1.2

Food	Amount	Calories	Total Fat (gm)	Saturated Fat (gm)
Baby foods—Vegetables *(cont'd)*				
Peas, strained	3.5 oz.	40	.3	0
Spinach, creamed	3.5 oz.	37	1.3	0
Squash	3.5 oz.	24	.2	0
Sweet potatoes	3.5 oz.	57	.1	0
Bacon, Canadian, broiled or fried, drained	2 slices (approx. 1 oz.)	25	.8	–
Bacon, cured, cooked	3 medium slices	109	9.3	3.3
Bagel Egg	1	230	2.5	.5
Plain	1	210	1.5	0
Bamboo shoots, raw	1 c.	41	.5	.1
Bananas, fresh	1 med.	105	.5	.2
Barbecue sauce	2 Tbsp.	60	trace	0
Barley, pearled, light, cooked	½ c.	95	.3	.1

Cholesterol (mg)	Sodium (mg)	Carbohydrates (gm)		Protein (gm)
		Total	Fiber	
0	4	8.1	1.2	3.5
0	48	5.7	.5	2.5
0	2	5.6	.7	.8
0	20	13.2	.6	1.1
10	345	.5	trace	5
16	301	.1	0	5.8
15	460	41	2.0	9.0
0	350	40	1.0	10.0
0	6	7.9	1.1	3.9
0	1	26.6	.6	1.1
0	330	14.0	0	0
0	2	21.7	.2	1.8

Food	Amount	Calories	Total Fat (gm)	Saturated Fat (gm)
Bass, striped, plain, cooked	3 oz.	122	3.9	.8
Beans, baked in tomato sauce with pork	½ c.	123	1.3	.5
Plain or vegetarian	½ c.	116	.6	.1
Beans, common, mature seeds, dry Kidney, canned, solids and liquid	1 c.	203	.8	.1
Pinto, calico, and red Mexican, cooked	1 c.	228	.8	.2
Others including black, brown, and bayo, cooked	1 c.	220	.8	.2
White, cooked	1 c.	232	.7	.2
Beans, lima (thin-seeded) Baby limas, frozen, cooked (thin-seeded), drained	1 c.	191	.5	.1
boiled, drained	1 c.	205	.5	.1

Cholesterol (mg)	Sodium (mg)	Carbohydrates (gm)		Protein (gm)
		Total	Fiber	
73	75	0	0	20.2
9	550	24.3	1.5	6.5
0	496	25.6	1.4	6.0
0	868	37.2	2.5	13.0
0	4	42.8	5.0	13.6
0	2	39.6	3.4	14.8
0	10	41.8	4.2	16.2
0	53	35.5	0	12.2
0	28	39.3	3.5	11.3

Food	Amount	Calories	Total Fat (gm)	Saturated Fat (gm)
Beans, lima *(cont'd)* canned, solids and liquids	1 c.	198	.5	.1
Fordhooks, frozen, and cooked (thick-seeded)	1 c.	166	.6	.1
Beans, mung, sprouted seeds, uncooked	1 c.	31	.2	.1
Beans, snap (includes Italian, yellow, and green) cooked	1 c.	44	.4	.1
frozen, cooked, and drained	1 c.	37	.1	trace
raw	1 c.	34	.1	trace
Beef Corned, cooked	3.5 oz.	209	15.8	5.3
Corned-beef hash, canned	1 c.	440	30	14
Flank steak, choice grade, braised	3 oz.	203	11.5	4.9

Cholesterol (mg)	Sodium (mg)	Carbohydrates (gm)		Protein (gm)
		Total	Fiber	
0	840	37.2	3.0	12.3
0	88	31.3	3.2	10.2
0	6	6.1	.8	3.1
0	4	9.9	1.8	2.4
0	19	8.7	1.4	2.0
0	7	7.9	1.2	2.0
82	945	0	0	15.2
100	840	23.0	2	19
59	60	0	0	23.3

Food	Amount	Calories	Total Fat (gm)	Saturated Fat (gm)
Beef *(cont'd)* Hamburger (ground beef) extra lean, cooked medium	3 oz.	213	13.5	5.3
lean, cooked medium	3 oz.	227	15.4	6.1
regular, cooked medium	3 oz.	241	17.2	6.8
Liver, cooked	3 oz.	134	4.1	1.6
Pot roast, choice grade, lean only	3 oz.	195	8.6	3.3
Round entire, choice grade, lean only	3 oz.	162	6.7	2.4
Round eye, choice grade, lean only	3 oz.	153	5.6	2.2
T bone steak, choice grade, lean only	3 oz.	178	8.7	3.5
Top round (London broil), choice grade, lean only	3 oz.	162	5.4	1.9

Cholesterol (mg)	Sodium (mg)	Carbohydrates (gm)		Protein (gm)
		Total	Fiber	
70	58	0	0	23.8
73	64	0	0	20.6
75	69	0	0	20.0
324	58	2.8	0	20.3
84	55	0	0	27.5
68	53	0	0	23.8
58	52	0	0	24.1
67	55	0	0	23.4
70	51	0	0	26.4

Food	Amount	Calories	Total Fat (gm)	Saturated Fat (gm)
Beef *(cont'd)* Whole ribs, choice grade, lean only	3 oz.	194	11.3	4.8
Beef stew, home recipe, with vegetables	1 c.	218	10.5	–
Beef stick, smoked (jerky)	1 stick	109	9.8	4.1
Beer. *See* **Beverages.**				
Beet greens, boiled, drained	1 c.	39	.3	trace
Beets boiled, drained	1 c.	73	.3	.1
canned, solids and liquid	1 c.	73	.3	trace
Beverages– Alcoholic and nonalcoholic carbonated/ noncarbonated. *See* individual fruits for fruit juices. *Alcoholic* Beer	12 oz.	146	0	0

Cholesterol (mg)	Sodium (mg)	Carbohydrates (gm)		Protein (gm)
		Total	Fiber	
68	58	0	0	21.7
–	91	15.2	–	15.7
26	293	1.1	0	4.3
0	344	7.9	1.6	3.7
0	128	16.7	1.3	2.8
0	658	17.0	1.5	2.0
0	18	31.2	0	1.1

Food	Amount	Calories	Total Fat (gm)	Saturated Fat (gm)
Beverages, alcoholic *(cont'd)*				
Beer, light (low-calorie) types	12 oz.	100	0	0
Gin, rum, vodka, whiskey	1 fl. oz.	73	0	0
Wines, table, all	4 oz.	82	0	0
Nonalcoholic, carbonated/ noncarbonated				
Club soda	12 oz.	0	0	0
Colas	12 oz.	152	0	0
Cream sodas	12 oz.	189	0	0
Diet sodas (with aspartame)	12 oz.	4	0	0
Fruit-flavored sodas	12 oz.	148	0	0
Fruit punch	12 oz.	195	0	0
Ginger ale	12 oz.	126	0	0

Cholesterol (mg)	Sodium (mg)	Carbohydrates (gm)		Protein (gm)
		Total	Fiber	
0	11	4.6	0	.7
0	.1	0	0	0
0	9	1.6	0	.2
0	75	0	0	0
0	15	38.5	0	0
0	44	49.3	0	0
0	21	.4	0	.4
0	41	38.5	0	0
0	30	45	0	0
0	26	32.2	0	0

Food	Amount	Calories	Total Fat (gm)	Saturated Fat (gm)
Beverages, nonalcoholic *(cont'd)* Lemonade, frozen, concentrated, diluted	12 oz.	114	.1	.1
Lemonade, powder	2 Tbsp.	150	0	trace
Root beer	12 oz.	152	0	0
Seltzer or sparkling water	12 oz.	0	0	0
Shake, fast food	12 oz.	438	12.8	7.9
Tonic water	12 oz.	125	0	0
Biscuits made from biscuit mix, with milk	2	190	6.5	2.8
with egg and sausage	1	587	39.1	15.1
Blackberries, boysenberries, dewberries, youngberries, fresh	1 c.	75	.6	0

Cholesterol (mg)	Sodium (mg)	Carbohydrates (gm)		Protein (gm)
		Total	Fiber	
0	12	29.1	0	trace
0	12	39.3	0	4.5
0	48	39.3	0	0
0	4	0	0	0
45	334	70.7	.3	11.7
0	15	32.6	0	0
3	384	30.0	1.8	2.0
305	1153	41.6	.2	19.5
0	0	18.5	5.9	1.04

Food	Amount	Calories	Total Fat (gm)	Saturated Fat (gm)
Black-eyed peas. *See* **Cowpeas and black-eyed peas.**				
Blueberries, fresh	1 c.	81	.6	0
Bluefish, cooked	3 oz.	103	3.5	.8
Boston brown bread	Approx. 1¼ oz.	102	.6	–
Bouillon cube. *See* **Soup.**				
Bran flakes 40% bran flakes	1 c.	126	.7	0
with raisins	1 c.	177	.3	0
Brazil nuts, dried, unblanched	1 oz.	187	18.9	4.6
Bread (average loaf) French or Vienna	1 slice	70	1	0
Italian	1 slice	70	1	0
Oatmeal/Oatbran	1 slice	60	1.0	0

Cholesterol (mg)	Sodium (mg)	Carbohydrates (gm)		Protein (gm)
		Total	Fiber	
0	9	20.5	1.9	1.0
49	50	0	0	16.7
—	121	220	.3	2.7
0	358	30.1	5.4	4.8
0	482	46.1	7.1	4.3
0	.6	3.7	.7	4.1
0	170	12.0	1.0	2.0
0	170	13.0	1.0	3.0
0	160	11.0	1.0	2.0

Food	Amount	Calories	Total Fat (gm)	Saturated Fat (gm)
Bread *(cont'd)* Potato	1 slice	80	1.0	0
Pumpernickel	1 slice	80	1.0	0
Raisin	1 slice	80	1.0	0
Rye	1 slice	80	.5	0
Stoneground, whole grain	1 slice	90	1	0
White enriched	1 slice	70	1.0	0
Whole wheat	1 slice	90	1.5	0
Bread crumbs, plain	¼ c.	120	1.5	0
Bread pudding	½ c.	210	7.4	2.9
Bread sticks	½ c.	200	9.8	1.8
Broccoli frozen, chopped, cooked	1 c.	56	.2	trace
raw	1 stalk	42	.6	.1

Cholesterol (mg)	Sodium (mg)	Carbohydrates (gm)		Protein (gm)
		Total	Fiber	
0	150	15.0	1.0	3.0
0	180	15.0	2.0	3.0
0	190	13.0	1.0	2.0
0	190	15.0	2.0	3.0
0	160	15.0	2.0	4.0
0	105	12.0	1.0	2.0
0	160	16.0	2.0	4.0
0	330	21.0	2.0	4.0
83	289	30.8	.4	6.5
0	744	24.0	1.2	3.0
0	48	10.8	2.4	6.2
0	41	7.9	1.7	4.5

Food	Amount	Calories	Total Fat (gm)	Saturated Fat (gm)
Broccoli *(cont'd)* whole stalks, fresh, cooked	1 stalk	47	.7	.1
Brussels sprouts, fresh, boiled	1 c.	65	.8	.2
Bulgur wheat, cooked	½ c.	75	.2	trace
Butter Light, salted	1 Tbsp.	50	6.0	4.0
Regular, salted	1 Tbsp.	100	11.0	7.0
Whipped, regular, salted	1 Tbsp.	60	7.0	5.0
Buttermilk, cultured, low fat, unsalted	1 c.	100	2.3	1.4

C

Food	Amount	Calories	Total Fat (gm)	Saturated Fat (gm)
Cabbage cooked, shredded	1 c.	33	.6	.1
raw, shredded	1 c.	18	.2	trace

Cholesterol (mg)	Sodium (mg)	Carbohydrates (gm)		Protein (gm)
		Total	Fiber	
0	43	8.5	1.8	5.0
0	35	14.5	2.3	4.3
0	5	16.9	.3	2.8
20	70	0	0	trace
30	85	0	0	0
20	75	0	0	0
10	125	12.0	0	8.3
0	12	6.7	.9	1.5
0	13	3.9	.9	1.0

Food	Amount	Calories	Total Fat (gm)	Saturated Fat (gm)
Cake *Commercial, packaged* Chocolate with chocolate icing	1 piece	310	14.0	4.5
Marble loaf, fat free	1 piece	130	0	0
Frozen, packaged Chocolate with chocolate icing	1 piece	250	13.0	11.0
Home recipe Plain	1 piece	313	120	–
Made from mix, as prepared Angel food	1 piece	140	0	0
Devil's food	1 piece	250	12.0	3.0
Gingerbread	1 piece	230	7.1	2.2
Marble	1 piece	250	11.0	2.0
Spice	1 piece	250	11.0	2.5
White	1 piece	240	10.0	2.5
Yellow	1 piece	250	10.0	2.5

Cholesterol (mg)	Sodium (mg)	Carbohydrates (gm)		Protein (gm)
		Total	Fiber	
20	290	46.0	2.0	3.0
0	190	29.0	1.0	2.0
25	180	33.0	2.0	3.0
—	258	48.1	—	3.9
0	270	31.0	trace	3.0
55	380	33.0	1.0	3.0
27	360	37.0	trace	2.0
45	270	36.0	.1	3.0
55	310	35.0	0	3.0
0	310	34.0	0	3.0
55	300	36.0	0	1.0

Food	Amount	Calories	Total Fat (gm)	Saturated Fat (gm)
Cake icings				
Dry mix				
Chocolate, prepared with butter	½ of package	159	5.5	1.0
Home recipe				
Chocolate, prepared with butter	½ of recipe	200	5.6	3.6
Ready-to-eat				
Chocolate	½ of package	153	6.8	2.1
Coconut	½ of package	159	9.2	2.7
Cream cheese	½ of package	159	6.7	1.9
Vanilla	½ of package	161	6.5	1.9
Candy				
Butterscotch	1 piece	24	.2	.1
Caramels	1 piece	31	.6	.5
chewing gum	1 stick	10	trace	0

Cholesterol (mg)	Sodium (mg)	Carbohydrates (gm)		Protein (gm)
		Total	Fiber	
10	63	29.8	0	.5
15	95	38.8	.2	.7
0	70	24.3	.2	.4
0	75	20.3	1.0	.6
0	13	25.6	.2	trace
0	35	26.7	.1	trace
1	3	5.7	0	trace
.6	20	6.2	0	.4
0	.2	2.9	0	0

Food	Amount	Calories	Total Fat (gm)	Saturated Fat (gm)
Candy *(cont'd)*				
Chocolate				
baking, squares, unsweetened	1 square (1 oz.)	149	15:8	9.3
bittersweet	1 oz.	136	9.8	5.2
semisweet	1 oz.	136	9.1	5.2
sweet (German)	1 oz.	132	7.7	4.4
Chocolate bars and commercial brands				
coconut center	1 small bar	72	4.3	2.3
fudge, caramel and peanuts	1 small bar	68	3.3	1.8
honeycombed hard candy, with peanut butter	1 small bar	91	3.9	1.8
milk, plain	1 (av. 1.5 oz.)	223	13.3	8.0
milk, with crisped rice	1 (av. 1.4 oz.)	198	10.6	6.4
milk, with nuts	1 (av. 1.5 oz.)	229	15.0	7.4

Cholesterol (mg)	Sodium (mg)	Carbohydrates (gm)		Protein (gm)
		Total	Fiber	
0	4	8.1	.7	2.9
0	0	15.6	.7	2.0
.3	0	16.3	.7	2.0
0	0	17.6	2.0	2.2
0	25	11.6	0	.7
0	40	9.0	.1	1.4
0	28	13.8	0	1.6
10	36	25.8	.2	3.0
8	58	25.4	.2	2.5
8	32	23.1	.7	3.9

Food	Amount	Calories	Total Fat (gm)	Saturated Fat (gm)
Candy *(cont'd)*				
mint	1 large pat	170	4.0	2.5
nougat and caramel	1 small bar	74	2.3	1.2
peanut butter cup	6 small	202	12.9	9.6
peanuts	10 pieces	208	13.4	5.8
raisins	10 pieces	41	1.6	.7
vanilla creams	3 pieces	200	11.0	6.0
Chocolate-flavored roll, chewy type	1 piece	22	.1	trace
Fudge, chocolate	1 piece	65	1.4	.9
Gumdrops	10 small	129	0	0
Jellybeans	10 small	40	.1	0
Licorice, lollipops/ hard candies	1 piece	23	0	0

Cholesterol (mg)	Sodium (mg)	Carbohydrates (gm) Total	Fiber	Protein (gm)
0	15	34.0	0	1.3
2	35	13.7	.1	.6
6.3	121	19.9	.4	4.6
4	16	19.8	0	5.2
trace	3.6	7.1	0	.5
5	60	25.0	1.0	2.0
0	0	5.2	0	.1
2	11	13.5	trace	.3
0	15	33.1	0	0
0	3	10.2	0	0
0	3	5.9	trace	0

Food	Amount	Calories	Total Fat (gm)	Saturated Fat (gm)
Candy *(cont'd)* Peanut bars	1 bar	209	13.4	1.7
Peanut brittle	1 oz.	129	5.5	1.4
Carrots fresh, cooked	1 c.	70	.3	trace
frozen, cooked	1 c.	51	.1	trace
raw	1 med.	31	.1	trace
Cashew nuts dry roasted	1 oz.	164	13.3	2.6
roasted in oil	1 oz.	165	13.8	2.7
Cauliflower, fresh, cooked	1 c.	29	.6	.1
Caviar, black lumpfish	1 Tbsp.	15	1.0	0
Celery fresh, diced, cooked, drained	1 c.	27	.3	.1
raw (8" x 1½" at root)	1 med. stalk	6	trace	trace

Cholesterol (mg)	Sodium (mg)	Carbohydrates (gm)		Protein (gm)
		Total	Fiber	
0	92	19.0	.8	6.2
4	129	19.8	.4	2.1
0	103	16.4	2.3	1.7
0	84	11.9	1.7	1.7
0	25	7.1	.7	.7
0	5	9	.2	4.4
0	5	8.1	.4	4.6
0	19	5.1	1.0	2.3
50	380	0	0	1.0
0	136	6.0	1.3	1.2
0	35	1.5	.3	.3

Food	Amount	Calories	Total Fat (gm)	Saturated Fat (gm)
Cereal. *See* **Bran flakes; Corn products; Granola; Oatmeal; Oats; Rice products; Wheat products**				
Chard, Swiss fresh, cooked, drained	1 c.	35	.2	0
raw	1 c.	7	.1	0
Cheese *Natural* Blue or Roquefort type	1 oz.	98	8.1	5.3
Brie (domestic)	1 oz.	93	7.7	—
Camembert (domestic)	1 oz.	83	6.7	4.3
Cheddar (domestic)	1 oz.	112	9.2	5.9
fat free	1 slice (¾ oz.)	30	0	0
reduced fat	1 oz.	70	4.5	3.0

Cholesterol (mg)	Sodium (mg)	Carbohydrates (gm)		Protein (gm)
		Total	Fiber	
0	314	7.2	1.6	3.3
0	76	1.3	.3	.6
21	388	.7	0	5.9
28	175	.1	0	5.8
20	233	.1	0	5.5
29	172	.4	0	6.9
5	290	3	0	5
10	200	1	0	8

Food	Amount	Calories	Total Fat (gm)	Salurated Fat (gm)
Cheese *(cont'd)*				
Cottage creamed or regular (4% milk fat)	½ c.	116	5.1	3.2
low fat (1% milk fat)	½ c.	81	1.2	.7
Cream fat free	1 oz.	29	0	0
light (neufchatel)	1 oz.	72	6.5	4.1
regular	1 oz.	97	9.7	6.1
Feta (domestic)	1 oz.	73	5.9	4.2
Mozzarella with part-skim milk	1 oz.	71	4.4	2.8
with whole milk	1 oz.	78	6.0	3.7
Parmesan, grated	1 Tbsp.	23	1.5	1.0
Provolone	1 oz.	98	7.4	4.7
Ricotta with part-skim milk	½ c.	171	9.8	6.1

Cholesterol (mg)	Sodium (mg)	Carbohydrates (gm)		Protein (gm)
		Total	Fiber	
17	458	3.0	0	14.1
5	459	3.1	0	14.0
3	144	2	0	4.0
21	111	.8	0	2.8
31	82	.7	0	2.1
25	310	1.1	0	3.9
16	129	.8	0	6.7
22	104	.6	0	5.4
4	93	.2	0	2.1
19	243	.6	0	7.1
38	155	6.4	0	14.1

Food	Amount	Calories	Total Fat (gm)	Saturated Fat (gm)
Cheese *(cont'd)* with whole milk	½ c.	216	16.1	10.3
Swiss	1 oz.	104	7.6	4.9
Pasteurized process American	1 oz.	104	8.7	5.5
Cheese food (American)	1 oz.	91	6.8	4.3
Cheese spread (American)	1 oz.	81	5.9	3.7
Pimiento (American)	1 oz.	104	8.7	5.4
Swiss, regular	1 oz.	93	6.9	4.4
Cheese puffs or twists	1 oz.	158	9.8	1.9
Cherries, maraschino	1 oz.	33	1.0	—
Cherries, sour canned, water pack	1 c.	88	.2	trace
fresh, red	1 c.	50	.3	.1

Cholesterol (mg)	Sodium (mg)	Carbohydrates (gm)		Protein (gm)
		Total	Fiber	
63	104	3.8	0	14.0
26	72	.9	0	7.9
26	397	.4	0	6.2
18	330	2.0	0	5.4
15	374	2.4	0	4.6
26	397	.5	trace	6.1
24	381	.6	0	6.9
1.1	300	15.4	.1	2.2
—	—	8.4	.1	.1
0	17	21.8	.2	1.9
0	3	12.2	.2	1.0

Food	Amount	Calories	Total Fat (gm)	Saturated Fat (gm)
Cherries, sweet canned, water pack	1 c.	115	.3	.1
fresh	1 c.	103	1.4	.3
Chestnuts, raw	1 oz.	64	.3	.1
Chicken Skinless, roasted Breast	½ breast	138	3.0	.8
Drumstick	1 drumstick	75	2.5	.7
Thigh	1 thigh	110	5.7	1.6
Wing	1 wing	43	1.7	.5
With skin, roasted Breast	½ breast	197	7.7	2.2
Drumstick	1 drumstick	114	5.9	1.6
Thigh	1 thigh	154	9.7	2.7
Wing	1 wing	100	6.7	1.9
Chicken, canned, with broth	3 oz.	138	6.7	1.8

Cholesterol (mg)	Sodium (mg)	Carbohydrates (gm)		Protein (gm)
		Total	Fiber	
0	3	29.5	.5	2.0
0	0	23.7	.6	1.7
0	.9	14.0	.5	1.2
71	62	0	0	25.8
40	41	0	0	12.3
50	46	0	0	13.7
18	19	0	0	6.4
84	71	0	0	29.2
48	47	0	0	14.2
58	53	0	0	15.6
29	28	0	0	9.3
–	419	0	0	18.2

Food	Amount	Calories	Total Fat (gm)	Saturated Fat (gm)
Chicken *(cont'd)* **Chicken,** fried	3 oz.	250	16.0	4.8
Chicken, liver, cooked	¼ c.	54	1.9	.6
Chicken chow mein, canned	7 oz.	60	2.5	1.0
Chicken fricassee	1 c.	386	22.3	–
Chicken nuggets	6 pieces	220	14.0	3.0
Chicken patties	1 patty	190	12.0	3.0
Chicken potpie, frozen	1 pie	550	34.0	7.0
Chickpeas, cooked	½ c.	137	2.2	.3
Chicory Greens, raw	1 c.	38	.5	.1
Head, bleached (Witloof)	½ c.	8	trace	trace
Chili, canned with beans	1 c.	220	7.0	1.5

Cholesterol (mg)	Sodium (mg)	Carbohydrates (gm)		Protein (gm)
		Total	Fiber	
50	40	14.0	0	14.0
218	17.6	.3	0	8.4
5	990	4.0	2.0	6.0
–	370	7.7	NA	36.7
36	480	11.0	0	13.0
30	230	11.0	1.0	10.0
45	630	43.0	5.0	19.0
0	6	22.8	2.1	7.4
0	75	7.8	1.3	2.8
0	1	1.8	0	.4
30	420	15.0	6.0	19.0

Food	Amount	Calories	Total Fat (gm)	Saturated Fat (gm)
Chocolate. *See* Candy.				
Chocolate and cocoa flavored beverage powder, regular	2–3 tsp.	76	.7	.4
Chocolate milk	8 oz.	208	8.5	5.3
Chocolate syrup	1 Tbsp.	41	.2	.1
Clams, cooked	3	123	1.7	.2
Coconut meat dried, sweetened, shredded	¼ c.	88	6.0	5.3
raw	2" x 2" piece	161	15.2	13.5
Cod, cooked	3 oz.	68	.6	.1
Coffee flavored, powdered	2 tsp.	62	2.1	1.8
regular or decaffeinated	1 c.	5	0	0

Cholesterol (mg)	Sodium (mg)	Carbohydrates (gm)		Protein (gm)
		Total	Fiber	
0	46	19.6	.2	.7
30	150	25.8	.2	8.0
0	18.1	11.1	trace	.4
56	93	4.3	0	21.3
0	47	8.8	.4	.6
0	9	6.9	2.0	1.5
36	45	0	0	14.8
0	99	10.8	0	.4
0	5	1	0	.3

Food	Amount	Calories	Total Fat (gm)	Saturated Fat (gm)
Cold cuts. *See* Luncheon meat and cold cuts.				
Coleslaw, cream	½ c.	41	1.5	.2
Collards, boiled, drained	1 c.	34	.3	0
Cookies *Made from mix, as prepared* Brownies	1	200	9.0	2.0
Chocolate chip	1	160	7.2	4.2
Packaged Animal crackers	14	140	4.0	1.0
Chocolate chip	3	160	8.0	2.5
Chocolate chip, reduced fat	3	150	6.0	1.5
Coconut bars	4	140	5.0	2.0
Fig bars	2	110	2.5	1.0
Gingersnaps	4	120	2.5	.5

Cholesterol (mg)	Sodium (mg)	Carbohydrates (gm)		Protein (gm)
		Total	Fiber	
5	14	7.3	.4	.8
0	20	7.6	.6	1.8
25	125	28.0	1.0	1.0
27	168	24.0	.5	2.0
0	135	24.0	trace	2.0
0	105	21.0	1.0	2.0
0	140	23.0	trace	2.0
0	130	20.0	1.0	2.0
0	120	20.0	1.0	1.0
0	170	22.0	trace	1.0

Food	Amount	Calories	Total Fat (gm)	Saturated Fat (gm)
Cookies *(cont'd)* Graham crackers, chocolate-covered	3	140	7.0	4.5
Graham crackers, plain	2 whole	120	3.5	.5
Oatmeal	1 large	80	3	.5
Oatmeal raisin	2	110	5	1.0
Sandwich-type Chocolate or vanilla, with cream filling	3	150	7.0	2.0
Chocolate with cream filling, reduced fat	3	140	5.0	1.0
Devil's food cookie cakes, fat free	1	50	0	0
Peanut butter	2	130	6.0	1.0
Shortbread	4	140	7.0	1.0
Sugar wafers, layered, with filling	5	140	7.0	1.5

Cholesterol (mg)	Sodium (mg)	Carbohydrates (gm)		Protein (gm)
		Total	Fiber	
0	105	19.0	trace	1.0
0	95	21.0	trace	1.0
0	65	12.0	trace	1.0
0	70	16.0	1.0	1.0
0	125	21.0	1.0	2.0
0	150	24.0	1.0	2.0
0	25	13.0	trace	1.0
trace	110	19.0	1.0	3.0
5	130	19.0	trace	2.0
0	15	20.0	trace	trace

Food	Amount	Calories	Total Fat (gm)	Saturated Fat (gm)
Cookies *(cont'd)*				
Vanilla wafers	8	140	5.0	1.0
Corn, sweet				
canned, cream style	1 c.	180	1.0	.2
canned, whole kernel, drained	1 c.	135	1.7	.3
fresh, cooked on the cob or kernels	1 med. ear or ½ c.	83	1	.2
frozen, on the cob, cooked	1 med. ear (corn only)	58	.4	.1
frozen, kernels, cooked, drained	1 c.	135	.2	trace
Corn bread				
home recipe, Southern style	1 piece	161	5.6	–
made from mix, as prepared	1 piece	180	5.6	1.6
Corn chips				
barbecue flavor	1 oz.	149	9.3	1.3

Cholesterol (mg)	Sodium (mg)	Carbohydrates (gm)		Protein (gm)
		Total	Fiber	
5	105	24.0	0	2.0
0	713	45.0	1.3	4.3
0	0	31.0	0	4.3
0	13	19.2	.5	2.5
0	3	13.9	.4	1.9
0	8	34.1	.8	5.0
—	490	22.7	—	5.8
30	320	30.0	1.3	2.0
0	218	16.1	.3	2.0

Food	Amount	Calories	Total Fat (gm)	Saturated Fat (gm)
Corn chips *(cont'd)* plain	1 oz.	154	9.5	1.3
Corn grits, cooked	1 c.	150	.5	.1
Corn products— Packaged, used mainly as ready-to-eat breakfast cereals Corn flakes plain	1 c.	110	0	0
sugar-coated	1 c.	156	0	0
Cornstarch	1 Tbsp.	29	trace	trace
Cowpeas and black-eyed peas cooked, drained	1 c.	162	.7	.2
Crab Alaskan king, cooked	3 oz.	81	1.3	.1
Blue, crab cakes	3.5 oz.	93	4.5	.9
Crabapple	1 c.	84	.3	.1
Crackers Animal. *See* Cookies.				

Cholesterol (mg)	Sodium (mg)	Carbohydrates (gm)		Protein (gm)
		Total	Fiber	
0	180	16.3	.3	1.9
0	0	32.5	.3	3.5
0	330	26.0	1.0	2.0
0	260	36.4	0	1.3
0	trace	7.0	0	trace
0	7	33.8	3.2	5.3
44	893	0	0	16.2
90	198	.3	trace	12.1
0	1	22.0	.7	.4

Food	Amount	Calories	Total Fat (gm)	Saturated Fat (gm)
Cheese	27 small	160	8.0	2.0
Classic golden	5	80	4.5	1.0
Classic golden, reduced fat	6	60	1.0	0
Classic golden, reduced salt	5	80	4.5	1.0
Graham. *See* Cookies.				
Rye wafers	2	60	0	0
Saltines	5	60	1.5	0
Sandwich-type, cheese, with peanut-butter filling	6	200	11.0	2.0
Thin wheat	16	140	6.0	1
Thin wheat, low salt	16	140	4.0	.5
Water cracker	5	45	0	0
Whole wheat	7	140	5.0	1.0

Cholesterol (mg)	Sodium (mg)	Carbohydrates (gm)		Protein (gm)
		Total	Fiber	
0	240	16.0	trace	4.0
0	150	9.0	trace	1.0
0	140	11.0	0	1.0
0	75	10.0	1.0	1.0
0	75	13.0	4.0	2.0
0	180	10.0	trace	2.0
0	420	22.0	1.0	4.0
0	120	20.0	2.0	3.0
23	85	23.0	1.0	2.0
0	90	9.0	1.0	2.0
0	170	21.0	4.0	3.0

Food	Amount	Calories	Total Fat (gm)	Saturated Fat (gm)
Cranberries, fresh	1 c.	47	.2	0
Cranberry juice cocktail	1 c.	145	.1	0
Cranberry-orange relish, uncooked	1 oz.	61	trace	0
Cranberry sauce, canned, strained sweetened	1 c.	378	.4	0
Cream Half and half	1 Tbsp.	20	1.7	1.1
Heavy, whipping, unwhipped	1 Tbsp.	51	5.5	3.4
Heavy, whipped, pressurized can	2 Tbsp.	20	1.5	1.0
Light, coffee or table	1 Tbsp.	29	2.9	1.8
Light, whipping, unwhipped	1 Tbsp.	44	4.6	2.9
Cream substitute powdered	1 tsp.	11	.7	.6

Cholesterol (mg)	Sodium (mg)	Carbohydrates (gm)		Protein (gm)
		Total	Fiber	
0	1	12.1	1.1	.4
0	10	37.2	0	.1
0	11	15.9	.2	.1
0	73	97.3	.8	.5
6	6	.6	0	.4
20	6	.4	0	.3
5	0	1.0	0	0
10	6	.6	0	.4
17	5	.5	0	.3
0	4	1.1	0	.1

Food	Amount	Calories	Total Fat (gm)	Saturated Fat (gm)
Cucumber	1 med. (7½" x 2")	40	.3	.1
Currants Black, European	3.5 oz.	32	.2	trace
Red and white	3.5 oz.	28	.1	trace
Custard, baked, egg, home recipe	1/2 c.	150	6.7	3.4

D

Food	Amount	Calories	Total Fat (gm)	Saturated Fat (gm)
Dandelion greens, raw	1 c.	25	.4	0
Dates	5	115	.2	0
Doughnuts reduced fat	1	220	6.0	1.5
regular, plain	1	170	9.0	4.0
Duck skinless, cooked	¼ duck	223	12.4	4.7
with skin, cooked	¼ duck	674	56.8	19.4

Cholesterol (mg)	Sodium (mg)	Carbohydrates (gm)		Protein (gm)
		Total	Fiber	
0	6	8.5	1.8	2.1
0	1	7.7	1.2	.7
0	1	6.9	1.7	.7
124	110	15.3	0	7.3
0	42	5.1	.9	1.5
0	1	30.6	.9	.8
15	270	40.0	trace	2.0
10	230	21.0	trace	3.0
99	72	0	0	26.1
168	118	0	0	38.0

Food	Amount	Calories	Total Fat (gm)	Saturated Fat (gm)

E

Food	Amount	Calories	Total Fat (gm)	Saturated Fat (gm)
Eel, cooked	3 oz.	197	12.5	2.5
Eggnog	1 c.	343	19	11.2
Eggplant, cooked	1 c.	28	.2	trace
Eggs fried in butter	1	83	6.4	2.4
hard- or soft-boiled, poached, raw	1	79	5.6	1.7
scrambled	1	93	5.8	2.8
white only, raw	1	16	trace	0
yolk only, raw	1	63	5.6	1.7
Egg substitute, liquid	2 oz. (1 egg)	53	2.1	.4
Endive (curly) and escarole, raw	1 c.	9	.1	trace

Cholesterol (mg)	Sodium (mg)	Carbohydrates (gm)		Protein (gm)
		Total	Fiber	
134	54	0	0	19.8
150	137	34.3	0	9.7
0	3	6.6	1.0	.8
246	144	.5	0	5.4
274	69	.6	0	6.1
243	151	1.3	0	5.8
0	51	.4	0	3.4
272	8	trace	0	2.8
1	112	.4	0	7.6
0	1	1.7	.5	.6

Food	Amount	Calories	Total Fat (gm)	Saturated Fat (gm)

F

Food	Amount	Calories	Total Fat (gm)	Saturated Fat (gm)
Farina, cooked	1 c.	117	.2	trace
Figs canned (light syrup pack), solids and liquid	½ c.	86	.1	trace
fresh	1 med.	37	.2	trace
Filberts (hazelnuts), dried, unblanched	1 oz.	181	17.9	1.3
Fish. *See* **individual names.**				
Fish sticks frozen, breaded	5 sticks	389	17.4	4.4
reduced fat, breaded	6 sticks	180	3.0	.5
Flatfish, cooked	3 oz.	98	1.3	.3
Flounder, cooked	3 oz.	98	1.3	.3
Frankfurters Beef	1 frank (⅛ lb.)	175	15.8	6.7

Cholesterol (mg)	Sodium (mg)	Carbohydrates (gm)		Protein (gm)
		Total	Fiber	
0	0	24.7	0	3.3
0	1	22.5	.8	.6
0	1	9.6	.6	.4
0	1	4.4	1.1	3.7
160	831	34.0	.6	22.4
25	440	26	0	13
57	88	0	0	20.2
57	88	0	1.3	20.2
34	570	1.0	0	6.7

Food	Amount	Calories	Total Fat (gm)	Saturated Fat (gm)
Frankfurters *(cont'd)*				
Beef, low fat	1 frank (⅛ lb.)	60	1.5	.5
Chicken/turkey	1 frank (⅛ lb.)	142	10.8	3.1
French toast, with butter	2 slices	377	20.0	8.1
Frozen fruit bars	1	63	.1	0
Frozen pudding pops	1	73	2.2	0
Fruit cocktail, canned, heavy syrup pack	½ c.	91	.1	trace
Fruit salad canned, heavy syrup pack	½ c.	91	.1	trace
canned, water pack	½ c.	38	.1	trace

G

Food	Amount	Calories	Total Fat (gm)	Saturated Fat (gm)
Garlic, raw	1 clove	5	trace	trace

Cholesterol (mg)	Sodium (mg)	Carbohydrates (gm)		Protein (gm)
		Total	Fiber	
20	480	5.0	0	7.0
56	660	1.0	0	7.2
123	543	38.1	.1	11.0
0	3	15.5	0	.9
0	79	12.1	trace	1.9
0	8	23.6	.6	.5
0	8	23.8	.8	.4
0	4	9.9	.8	.5
0	1	1	trace	.2

Food	Amount	Calories	Total Fat (gm)	Saturated Fat (gm)
Gelatin desserts, made with water; reduced calorie, sweetened with aspartame	1 c.	16	0	0
regular	1 c.	159	0	0
Goose skinless, cooked	⅟₁₆ goose	170	9.1	3.3
with skin, cooked	⅟₁₆ goose	305	21.9	6.8
Granola, packaged with almonds and seeds	⅓ c.	220	9.0	1.0
Granola bars hard, plain	1 oz. bar	135	5.7	.7
soft, low fat	1 oz. bar	110	2.0	0
soft, plain, uncoated	1 oz. bar	127	4.9	2.1
Grapefruit canned, light syrup pack	½ c.	75	.1	trace
fresh—white, pink, or red	½ med.	40	.1	trace

Cholesterol (mg)	Sodium (mg)	Carbohydrates (gm)		Protein (gm)
		Total	Fiber	
0	112	1.6	0	0
0	114	37.8	0	3.2
69	54	0	0	20.7
91	70	0	0	25.1
0	85	29.0	4.0	6.0
0	84	18.4	.3	2.9
0	65	21.0	1.0	2.0
.3	79	19.2	.3	2.1
0	3	19.3	.4	.8
0	0	10.1	.3	.8

Food	Amount	Calories	Total Fat (gm)	Saturated Fat (gm)
Grapefruit juice canned, sweetened	1 c.	115	.3	trace
canned, unsweetened	1 c.	95	.3	trace
fresh—white, pink, or red	1 c.	98	.3	trace
frozen concentrate, unsweetened, diluted per directions	1 c.	103	.3	trace
Grape juice canned or bottled	1 c.	153	.2	.1
frozen concentrate, sweetened, diluted per directions	1 c.	128	.2	.1
Grapes American type (Concord, Delaware, Niagara, Catawba, scuppernong), fresh	1 c.	58	.3	.1
canned, heavy syrup pack	1 c.	182	.2	.1
European type, fresh	1 c.	118	1.0	.3

Cholesterol (mg)	Sodium (mg)	Carbohydrates (gm)		Protein (gm)
		Total	Fiber	
0	5	27.8	0	1.5
0	3	22.5	0	1.3
0	3	23.0	0	1.3
0	3	24.3	0	1.4
0	8	37.5	.8	1.5
0	5	32	.3	.5
0	2	15.9	.7	.6
0	13	49.2	.5	1.3
0	3.3	29.7	.8	1.2

Food	Amount	Calories	Total Fat (gm)	Saturated Fat (gm)
Gravy canned, for turkey	¼ c.	30	1.2	.3
dry mix, for turkey, as prepared	¼ c.	20	0	0
Grits. *See* **Corn grits.**				
Guavas	1	46	.5	.2
Guinea hen, flesh and skin, raw	¼ hen	362	18.6	5.4

H

Food	Amount	Calories	Total Fat (gm)	Saturated Fat (gm)
Haddock, cooked	3 oz.	93	.8	.2
Halibut, cooked	3 oz.	116	2.4	.3
Ham. *See* **Pork.**				
Hamburger. *See* **Beef.**				
Herring, pickled	3 pieces	119	8.2	1.1
Hickory nuts, dried	1 oz.	188	18.4	2.0

Cholesterol (mg)	Sodium (mg)	Carbohydrates (gm)		Protein (gm)
		Total	Fiber	
1	290	3	–	1.5
0	270	4.0	0	1.0
0	2.7	10.9	5.1	.7
–	88	0	0	45.4
61	73	0	0	20.2
34	58	0	0	22.3
6	395	4.4	0	6.5
0	.3	5.2	.9	3.6

Food	Amount	Calories	Total Fat (gm)	Saturated Fat (gm)
Hollandaise. *See* Sauces.				
Hominy grits. *See* Corn grits.				
Honey	1 Tbsp.	63	0	0
Horseradish	1 Tbsp.	0	0	0

I

Food	Amount	Calories	Total Fat (gm)	Saturated Fat (gm)
Ice cream and frozen custard regular (approximately 10% fat)	½ c.	135	7.2	4.5
rich (approximately 16% fat)	½ c.	174	11.9	7.4
soft-serve, french vanilla	½ c.	188	11.2	6.7
Ice milk hard	½ c.	92	12.6	1.8
soft-serve	½ c.	112	2.3	1.4
fat free	½ c.	90	0	0

Cholesterol (mg)	Sodium (mg)	Carbohydrates (gm)		Protein (gm)
		Total	Fiber	
0	1	17.2	0	.1
0	120	2.4	0	0
30	58	15.9	0	2.4
44	54	16.0	0	2.1
77	77	19.0	0	3.5
9	52	14.4	0	2.6
7	82	19.2	0	4.0
0	105	20.0	0	4.0

Food	Amount	Calories	Total Fat (gm)	Saturated Fat (gm)
Ice milk *(cont'd)* fat free, no sugar added	½ c.	70	0	0
Ices, water	½ c.	77	0	0
Icing. *See* **Cake icings.**				

J

Jams and preserves	1 Tbsp.	48	trace	trace
Jellies	1 Tbsp.	51	trace	trace
Jerusalem artichokes, raw	1 c.	113	trace	0

K

Kale, cooked	1 c.	42	.5	.1
Ketchup. *See* **Tomato catsup.**				
Kiwi	1 med.	47	.3	0
Kumquats, fresh	3 small	36	.1	0

Cholesterol (mg)	Sodium (mg)	Carbohydrates (gm) Total	Fiber	Protein (gm)
0	45	18	0	4.0
0	0	32	0	.4
0	8	12.9	.1	.1
0	7	13.3	.1	.1
0	0	26.0	1.2	3.0
0	30	.6	1.0	2.5
0	4	11.5	.8	.8
0	3	9.4	2.1	.5

Food	Amount	Calories	Total Fat (gm)	Saturated Fat (gm)

L

Food	Amount	Calories	Total Fat (gm)	Saturated Fat (gm)
Lake herring (cisco), smoked	3 oz.	148	9.9	1.4
Lake trout. *See* **Trout**				
Lamb Cubes, for stew, lean only, cooked	3 oz.	155	6.1	2.2
Ground, cooked	3 oz.	236	16.4	6.8
Leg, choice grade, lean only, cooked	3 oz.	159	6.4	2.3
Loin, choice grade, lean only, cooked	3 oz.	168	8.2	3.1
Shoulder, choice grade, lean only, cooked	3 oz.	170	9.0	3.4
Lard	1 Tbsp.	116	12.8	5.0
Leeks, raw	2	153	.8	.1
Lemon juice, canned or bottled, unsweetened	1 c.	53	.8	.1

Cholesterol (mg)	Sodium (mg)	Carbohydrates (gm)		Protein (gm)
		Total	Fiber	
27	401	0	0	13.7
75	63	0	0	23.4
81	68	0	0	20.7
74	57	0	0	23.6
73	55	0	0	22.2
73	57	0	0	20.8
12	trace	0	0	0
0	50	35.3	3.8	3.8
0	53	16.3	0	1.0

Food	Amount	Calories	Total Fat (gm)	Saturated Fat (gm)
Lemon juice *(cont'd)* fresh	1 c.	63	0	0
Lemonade. *See* **Beverages.**				
Lemons, fresh, peeled	1 med.	17	.2	trace
Lentils, cooked	1 c.	232	.8	.1
Lettuce Butterhead varieties	1 head (4" diam.)	22	.4	.1
Iceberg	1 head	68	1.1	.2
Loose-leafed, Romaine	2 large leaves	4	.1	trace
Lime juice, fresh, canned, or bottled, unsweetened	1 c.	68	.3	trace
Limeade, concentrate, diluted	1 c.	103	0	trace
Limes, fresh	1 med.	20	.1	trace

Cholesterol (mg)	Sodium (mg)	Carbohydrates (gm)		Protein (gm)
		Total	Fiber	
0	3	21.5	0	1.0
0	1	5.5	.2	.6
0	4	40	5.6	18.4
0	8	3.8	0	2.2
0	47	11.1	2.6	5.2
0	2	.7	.1	.3
0	3	22.5	0	1.0
0	5	27.5	0	0
0	1	7.0	.3	.5

Food	Amount	Calories	Total Fat (gm)	Saturated Fat (gm)
Liver. *See* **Beef** or **Chicken.**				
Lobster, cooked	3 oz.	82	.5	.1
Loganberries, frozen	1 c.	79	.4	0
Luncheon meat and cold cuts Bologna, beef	1 slice (1 oz.)	89	8.1	3.5
Bologna, light	1 slice (1 oz.)	50	4.0	1.5
Chicken roll	1 slice (1 oz.)	45	2.1	.6
Ham, chopped, canned	1 oz.	68	5.4	1.8
Ham, regular	1 slice (1 oz.)	52	3.0	1.0
Liverwurst	1 slice (⅔ oz.)	58	5.1	1.9
Olive loaf	1 slice (1 oz.)	67	4.7	1.7

Cholesterol (mg)	Sodium (mg)	Carbohydrates (gm)		Protein (gm)
		Total	Fiber	
60	317	1.1	0	17.1
0	1	18.6	0	2.1
17	280	.2	0	3.5
15	310	1.0	0	3.0
14	167	.7	0	5.6
14	390	.1	0	4.6
16	376	.9	0	5.0
28	—	.4	0	4.6
11	424	2.6	0	3.4

Food	Amount	Calories	Total Fat (gm)	Saturated Fat (gm)
Luncheon meats and cold cuts *(cont'd)* Pastrami	1 slice (1 oz.)	43	2.3	1.0
Salami, beef	1 slice (⅔ oz.)	59	4.7	2.0
Turkey or chicken breast	1 slice (⅔ oz.)	23	.3	.1
Turkey bologna	1 slice (1 oz.)	57	4.3	–
Turkey ham	1 slice (1 oz.)	37	1.5	.5
Turkey pastrami	1 slice (1 oz.)	40	1.8	.5
Turkey salami	1 slice (1 oz.)	56	3.9	–

M

Food	Amount	Calories	Total Fat (gm)	Saturated Fat (gm)
Macadamia nuts, dried	1 oz.	200	21.1	3.1
Macaroni. *See* **Pasta.**				

Cholesterol (mg)	Sodium (mg)	Carbohydrates (gm)		Protein (gm)
		Total	Fiber	
16.7	320	0	0	5.3
14	269	.6	0	3.4
9	298	0	0	4.7
28	251	.3	0	3.9
–	285	.1	0	5.4
–	298	.5	0	5.3
23	287	.2	0	4.7
0	1.4	3.9	1.5	2.4

Food	Amount	Calories	Total Fat (gm)	Saturated Fat (gm)
Mackerel, Atlantic, cooked	3 oz.	218	14.8	3.5
Mangoes, fresh	1 small	135	.6	.1
Margarine Canola, nonfat, soft tub	1 Tbsp.	20	2.0	0
Corn, regular, stick or soft tub	1 Tbsp.	101	11.3	20
Soybean, reduced fat, stick or soft tub	1 Tbsp.	50	6.0	1.0
Marmalade	1 Tbsp.	49	0	0
Mayonnaise. *See* **Salad dressings**				
Melons, fresh Cantaloupe	½ melon	88	.8	0
Casaba	⅒ melon	43	.2	0
Honeydew	⅒ melon	44	.1	0

Cholesterol (mg)	Sodium (mg)	Carbohydrates (gm)		Protein (gm)
		Total	Fiber	
63	69	0	0	19.9
0	4	35.4	1.7	1.0
0	105	0	0	0
0	140 (av.)	.1	0	.1
0	50	0	0	.1
0	11	13.3	0	.1
0	23	21.0	1.0	2.2
0	20	10.3	.8	1.5
0	13	11.5	.8	.6

Food	Amount	Calories	Total Fat (gm)	Saturated Fat (gm)
Milk, cow's				
Canned condensed, sweetened	½ c.	491	13.4	8.4
evaporated, unsweetened	½ c.	169	9.6	5.6
evaporated, skimmed (less than ¼ of 1% butterfat)	½ c.	100	.3	.2
Chocolate beverages. *See* Chocolate milk.				
Dry skim, nonfat solids (instant)	1 c.	244	.5	.3
skim, nonfat solids (regular)	1 c.	434	.9	.6
whole	1 c.	635	34.2	21.4
Malted, powder	3 heaping tsp.	86	1.6	.9
Pasteurized and raw low fat (1% fat)	1 c.	102	2.6	1.6

Cholesterol (mg)	Sodium (mg)	Carbohydrates (gm)		Protein (gm)
		Total	Fiber	
52	195	83	0	12.1
37	134	12.6	0	8.6
5	147	14.5	0	9.7
12	374	35.5	0	24.9
24	642	62.4	0	43.4
124	460	49.2	0	33.7
4.2	102	15.8	0	2.3
10	122	11.7	0	8.0

Food	Amount	Calories	Total Fat (gm)	Saturated Fat (gm)
Milk, cow's *(cont'd)* low fat (2% fat)	1 c.	122	4.6	2.9
skim	1 c.	86	.4	.3
whole (3.3% fat)	1 c.	484	8.1	5.1
See also Buttermilk; Yogurt				
Milk, goat's	1 c.	168	10.1	6.5
Milk, human	1 c.	172	10.8	4.9
Molasses	1 Tbsp.	53	trace	0
Muffins, enriched flour commercial, fat free	1	120	0	0
home recipe, blueberry	1	112	3.7	–
made from mix, with egg, milk	1	140	5.0	1.0
Mushrooms, cultivated commercially, canned, drained	½ c.	19	.2	trace

Cholesterol (mg)	Sodium (mg)	Carbohydrates (gm)		Protein (gm)
		Total	Fiber	
20	122	11.7	0	8.1
5	127	11.9	0	8.4
34	120	11.4	0	8.1
27	122	10.9	0	8.7
34	42	17.0	0	2.5
0	7	13.8	0	0
0	220	26.0	trace	2.0
–	253	16.8	–	2.9
20	220	29.0	0	2.0
0	0	3.8	0	1.5

Food	Amount	Calories	Total Fat (gm)	Saturated Fat (gm)
Mushrooms *(cont'd)* fresh	½ c.	9	.1	trace
Mussels, cooked	3 oz.	143	3.8	.8
Mustard, prepared	1 tsp.	0	0	0
Mustard greens, cooked	1 c.	21	.3	trace

N

Food	Amount	Calories	Total Fat (gm)	Saturated Fat (gm)
Nectarines, fresh	1 med.	66	.7	0
Nuts. *See* individual names.				

O

Food	Amount	Calories	Total Fat (gm)	Saturated Fat (gm)
Oatmeal instant, maple-flavored, cooked	1 c.	380	4.0	0
oatmeal/rolled oats, cooked	1 c.	144	2.3	.5
Oats, flaked	1 c.	156	2.0	.8
Ocean perch. *See* Perch.				

Cholesterol (mg)	Sodium (mg)	Carbohydrates (gm) Total	Fiber	Protein (gm)
0	2	1.6	.3	.7
47	308	6.2	0	19.8
0	55	0	0	0
0	23	3.0	1.0	3.3
0	0	15.9	.6	1.2
0	0	72.0	6.0	12.0
0	2	25.1	.5	6.0
0	247	32.5	1.3	2.6

Food	Amount	Calories	Total Fat (gm)	Saturated Fat (gm)
Oils, salad or cooking Canola	1 Tbsp.	130	13.5	1.0
Corn	1 Tbsp.	119	13.5	1.7
Olive	1 Tbsp.	119	13.5	1.8
Other vegetables (safflower, sunflower)	1 Tbsp.	119	13.5	1.2
Okra, cooked	10 pods (3" x ⅝")	36	.2	.1
Olives canned, ripe, small	3	15	1.4	.2
jumbo, supercolossal	3	37	3.1	.4
Onion powder	1 tsp.	7	trace	0
Onions, mature boiled	½ c.	46	.2	trace
raw	½ c.	30	.1	trace
Orange drink, powder	1 Tbsp.	92	trace	trace

Cholesterol (mg)	Sodium (mg)	Carbohydrates (gm)		Protein (gm)
		Total	Fiber	
0	0	0	0	0
0	0	0	0	0
0	trace	0	0	0
0	0	0	0	0
0	6	8.0	1.0	2.1
0	114	.8	0	.1
0	408	2.5	0	.5
0	1	1.7	.1	.2
0	3	10.7	.7	1.5
0	2	6.9	.5	1.0
0	4	23.5	0	trace

Food	Amount	Calories	Total Fat (gm)	Saturated Fat (gm)
Orange juice canned	1 c.	105	.3	.1
chilled	1 c.	110	.8	.1
fresh	1 c.	113	.5	.1
frozen concentrate, diluted per directions	1 c.	113	.2	trace
Oranges, fresh, peeled, no seeds All typical varieties	1 med.	62	.1	trace
California navels (winter)	1 med.	66	.1	trace
California Valencias (summer)	1 med.	59	.4	trace
Florida (typical varieties)	1 med.	70	.3	trace
Oysters, cooked	6 oysters	57	2.0	.6

Cholesterol (mg)	Sodium (mg)	Carbohydrates (gm)		Protein (gm)
		Total	Fiber	
0	5	25.0	.3	1.5
0	3	25.0	0	2.0
0	3	26.0	.3	1.8
0	3	27.0	.1	1.8
0	0	15.5	.5	1.2
0	1	16.6	.7	1.4
0	0	14.3	.6	1.2
0	0	17.4	.5	1.1
44	176	3.3	0	5.9

Food	Amount	Calories	Total Fat (gm)	Saturated Fat (gm)

P

Food	Amount	Calories	Total Fat (gm)	Saturated Fat (gm)
Pancakes and waffles made from mix, as prepared	2 cakes	170	6.0	1.5
made from mix, reduced fat, as prepared	2 cakes	150	2.5	.5
Papayas, fresh	1 fruit	130	.5	.1
Parsley, raw, chopped	1 Tbsp.	4	.1	0
Parsnips, cooked	1 c.	135	.5	.1
Pasta cooked	1 c.	201	1.0	.1
egg, cooked	1 c.	222	2.5	.5
spinach, cooked	1 c.	186	.9	.1
Pastina, egg	2 oz.	210	2.5	1.0
Peaches canned, heavy syrup pack	½ c.	93	.1	trace

Cholesterol (mg)	Sodium (mg)	Carbohydrates (gm)		Protein (gm)
		Total	Fiber	
0	490	25.0	trace	3.0
0	460	27.0	trace	3.0
0	10	32.7	2.7	2.0
0	6	.7	.1	.3
0	17	32.5	3.7	2.2
0	1	40.4	.1	6.9
55	12	41.3	.2	8.0
0	20	37.4	1.7	6.6
70	15	38.0	2.0	10.0
0	8	25.0	.4	.6

Food	Amount	Calories	Total Fat (gm)	Saturated Fat (gm)
Peaches *(cont'd)* canned, light syrup pack	½ c.	68	trace	trace
fresh	1 med.	37	.1	trace
Peanut butter (moderate amounts of fat, sweetener, and salt)	1 Tbsp.	93	7.9	1.5
Peanuts, unroasted, unsalted	1 oz.	163	13.8	1.9
Pears canned, heavy syrup pack	½ c.	93	.2	trace
canned, light syrup pack	½ c.	71	trace	trace
fresh, with skin	1 med.	98	.7	trace
Peas canned, cooked, drained	1 c.	115	.6	.1
fresh, cooked, drained	1 c.	140	.4	.1
frozen, cooked, drained	1 c.	130	.5	.1

Cholesterol (mg)	Sodium (mg)	Carbohydrates (gm)		Protein (gm)
		Total	Fiber	
0	6	18.3	.4	.6
0	0	9.7	.5	.6
0	76	3.3	.4	3.9
0	2 (salted, 226)	6.0	1.4	6.6
0	6	24.8	.8	.3
0	6	19	.8	.3
0	0	25.2	2.3	.7
0	365	21.0	3.3	7.3
0	5	26.0	3.8	9.0
0	145	23.8	3.5	8.6

Food	Amount	Calories	Total Fat (gm)	Saturated Fat (gm)
Pecans, dried	1 oz.	191	19.3	1.5
Pepperoni. *See* **Sausage**				
Peppers Hot chili, canned, cooked	½ c.	17	.1	trace
Hot chili, raw	1 pepper	18	.1	trace
Sweet, raw	½ c.	14	.1	trace
Perch, cooked	3 oz.	98	1.0	.2
Persimmons	1 small	117	.3	0
Pheasant, flesh only, uncooked	¼ pheasant	222	6.0	2.0
Pickle relish, sweet	1 Tbsp.	19	.1	trace
Pickles Dill	1 large (65 g)	12	.1	trace
Sour	1 medium (35 g)	4	.1	trace

Cholesterol (mg)	Sodium (mg)	Carbohydrates (gm)		Protein (gm)
		Total	Fiber	
0	.3	5.2	.5	2.2
0	0	6.1	.8	.6
0	3	4.3	.8	.9
0	1	3.2	.2	.4
96	66	0	0	20.8
0	2	31.0	2.5	1.0
–	62	0	0	39.3
0	121	5.2	.1	.1
0	855	2.7	.4	.4
0	417	.8	.2	.1

Food	Amount	Calories	Total Fat (gm)	Saturated Fat (gm)
Pickles *(cont'd)*				
Sweet	1 large (35 g)	40	.1	trace
Pies (1 piece equals approx. ⅙ of a 9" pie.)				
Apple	1 piece	300	14.0	3.5
Boston cream	1 piece	170	5.0	1.0
Chocolate cream	1 piece	290	14.0	4.0
Coconut custard	1 piece	280	12.0	5.0
Lemon meringue	1 piece	270	6.0	1.0
Mince	1 piece	320	13.6	–
Pecan	1 piece	431	23.6	–
Pigs' feet, pickled	3 oz.	169	13.4	4.7
Pike, cooked	3 oz.	94	.8	.1
Pimientos, canned	1 Tbsp.	3	trace	trace

Cholesterol (mg)	Sodium (mg)	Carbohydrates (gm)		Protein (gm)
		Total	Fiber	
0	324	11.0	.2	.1
0	300	42.0	2.0	2.0
25	140	29.0	0	2.0
0	180	37.0	1.0	2.0
75	350	35.0	0	7.9
45	290	51.0	1.0	3.0
–	529	48.6	–	3.0
–	228	52.8	–	5.3
77	–	trace	0	11.3
42	41	0	0	20.6
0	2	.6	.1	.1

Food	Amount	Calories	Total Fat (gm)	Saturated Fat (gm)
Pineapple canned, heavy syrup pack	2 slices	91	.1	trace
canned, light syrup pack	2 slices	60	.1	trace
fresh, diced	1 c.	75	.6	trace
Pineapple and grapefruit juice drink, canned	1 c.	118	.3	trace
Pineapple juice, canned, unsweetened	1 c.	140	.2	trace
Pistachio nuts, dry roasted	1 oz.	173	15.1	1.9
Pita bread regular size	1 (approx. 2 oz.)	150	1.0	0
small size	1 (approx. 1 oz.)	70	0	0
Pizza, baked	⅛ of a 12" pie			

Cholesterol (mg)	Sodium (mg)	Carbohydrates (gm)		Protein (gm)
		Total	Fiber	
0	1	23.5	.5	.4
0	1	15.7	.5	.4
0	2	19.1	.8	.6
0	35	29.0	0	.2
0	3	34.5	.3	.8
0	2	7.9	.5	4.3
0	290	31.0	1.0	6.0
0	140	15.0	trace	3.0

Food	Amount	Calories	Total Fat (gm)	Saturated Fat (gm)
Pizza *(cont'd)* with cheese	1 slice	139	3.2	1.6
with meat and vegetables	1 slice	185	5.4	1.5
Plate dinners— **Frozen, packaged.** **Note: Varies** **greatly by brand.** Beef tips with gravy, noodles, seasoned vegetables, and dessert	16 oz.	450	16.0	6.0
Chicken, rice, vegetables, and dessert, reduced calorie	12 oz.	270	4	1.5
Chicken, roasted, with mashed potatoes and mixed vegetables	14 oz.	670	42.0	15.0
Fish, fried, with potatoes, seasoned vegetables, and dessert	10 oz.	500	20.0	15.0
Plums canned, heavy syrup pack	½ c.	111	.1	trace

Cholesterol (mg)	Sodium (mg)	Carbohydrates (gm)		Protein (gm)
		Total	Fiber	
10	333	20.3	.3	7.6
21	384	21.4	.8	13.1
120	870	49.0	9.0	28.0
35	340	40.0	6.0	20.0
205	2100	32.0	7.0	43.0
90	1030	59.0	6.0	19.0
0	24	28.7	.4	.5

Food	Amount	Calories	Total Fat (gm)	Saturated Fat (gm)
Plums *(cont'd)* fresh	1 med.	37	.4	trace
Pollack, cooked	3 oz.	98	1.1	.1
Pomegrantes, fresh	1 med.	105	.5	0
Popcorn air-popped	1 c.	31	.3	trace
caramel	1 c.	154	4.6	1.3
microwave, low fat	1 c.	23	1.0	trace
microwave, regular	1 c.	33	2.0	.7
oil-popped	1 c.	55	3.1	.5
Pork Boston blade, fresh, roasted, lean only	3 oz.	213	14.0	4.8
Ham, canned, roasted, extra lean	3 oz.	113	4.1	1.3
Ham, cured, fresh, whole, roasted	3 oz.	131	4.6	1.5

Cholesterol (mg)	Sodium (mg)	Carbohydrates (gm)		Protein (gm)
		Total	Fiber	
0	0	8.9	.4	.5
76	92	0	0	20.8
0	5	26.2	.3	1.5
0	trace	6.2	.3	1.0
0	74	28.2	.6	1.4
0	53	4.0	0	.7
0	60	4.0	0	.7
0	97	6.3	.4	1.0
82	61	0	0	20.3
25	946	.4	0	17.7
46	1106	0	0	20.9

Food	Amount	Calories	Total Fat (gm)	Saturated Fat (gm)
Pork *(cont'd)* Ham steak, boneless, fresh, extra lean	3 oz.	102	3.6	1.2
Loin, fresh, roasted, lean only	3 oz.	200	11.5	4.0
Sirloin, fresh, roasted, lean only	3 oz.	196	11.0	3.8
Spare ribs, fresh, lean and fat, cooked	3 oz.	331	25.3	9.8
Pork and beans. *See* **Beans, common.**				
Potato chips barbecue flavor	1 oz.	140	9.3	2.3
plain	1 oz.	153	9.9	3.1
reduced-fat varieties	1 oz.	150	10.0	3.0
reduced-salt varieties	1 oz.	130	6.0	1.0

Cholesterol (mg)	Sodium (mg)	Carbohydrates (gm)		Protein (gm)
		Total	Fiber	
38	1058	0	0	16.3
75	58	0	0	22.4
75	52	0	0	22.9
101	78	0	0	24.3
0	214	15.1	.5	2.2
0	170	15.1	.5	2.0
0	85	14.0	1.0	2.0
0	140	17.0	1.0	2.0

Food	Amount	Calories	Total Fat (gm)	Saturated Fat (gm)
Potatoes, white baked or microwaved, with skin	1 med. (202 g.)	218	.2	trace
boiled, with skin	1 med. (136 g.)	119	.1	trace
canned, drained	1 c.	109	.4	.1
chips	1 oz.	153	9.9	3.1
dehydrated mashed (flakes), as prepared before adding milk and fat	1 c.	160	8.0	1.5
french-fried, frozen, heated in oven	10 pieces	111	4.4	2.2
french-fried, in vegetable oil	10 pieces	158	8.3	2.5
Pretzels, hard, plain	1 oz.	109	1.0	.2
Prune juice	1 c.	178	.1	trace

Cholesterol (mg)	Sodium (mg)	Carbohydrates (gm)		Protein (gm)
		Total	Fiber	
0	16	50.5	1.3	4.6
0	5	27.5	.4	2.6
0	0	24.7	.5	2.5
0	170	15.1	.5	2.0
5	460	19.0	1.0	3.0
0	15	16.9	.4	1.8
0	108	19.8	.4	2.0
0	490	22.6	.1	2.6
0	10	43.8	trace	1.5

Food	Amount	Calories	Total Fat (gm)	Saturated Fat (gm)
Prunes dried, cooked, no sugar added	1 c.	213	.4	trace
dried, softened, uncooked	1 c.	398	.8	.1
Puddings dry mix, instant, made with 2% milk	½ c.	146	2.7	1.6
dry mix, instant, sugar free, made with skim milk	½ c.	70	0	0
dry mix, regular, made with 2% milk	½ c.	151	2.9	1.7
Pumpkin, canned	1 c.	85	.8	.3
Pumpkin and squash seed kernels, roasted	1 oz.	127	5.5	1.1

Q

Food	Amount	Calories	Total Fat (gm)	Saturated Fat (gm)
Quail, flesh and skin, uncooked	½ quail	107	6.7	1.9

Cholesterol (mg)	Sodium (mg)	Carbohydrates (gm)		Protein (gm)
		Total	Fiber	
0	4	59.6	1.9	2.6
0	7	105	3.3	4.3
9	406	27.0	.1	4.4
0	330	12.0	0	0
10	150	28.1	.3	4.7
0	13	20.3	4.0	2.8
0	5	15.4	10.3	5.3
—	29	0	0	10.9

Food	Amount	Calories	Total Fat (gm)	Saturated Fat (gm)
R				
Rabbit, cooked	3 oz.	144	2.9	.9
Radishes, raw	4	3	.1	trace
Raisins, uncooked	1 c. pressed down	503	.8	.3
Raspberries fresh	1 c.	61	.7	trace
frozen, sweetened	1 c.	258	.4	trace
Relish. *See* **Pickle relish.**				
Rhubarb frozen, cooked, sugar added	½ c.	140	.1	0
uncooked	1 c.	26	.2	0
Rice Brown, cooked	1 c.	222	1.8	.4
Instant, cooked	1 c.	163	.3	trace

Cholesterol (mg)	Sodium (mg)	Carbohydrates (gm)		Protein (gm)
		Total	Fiber	
103	38	0	0	27.5
0	4	.6	.1	.1
0	20	132.5	2.3	5.7
0	0	14.5	3.8	1.1
0	3	65.5	5.5	1.8
0	1	37.6	1.0	.5
0	5	5.5	.9	1.1
0	10	46.0	.7	5.2
0	5	35.5	.2	3.5

Food	Amount	Calories	Total Fat (gm)	Saturated Fat (gm)
Rice *(cont'd)* White, enriched, regular, cooked	1 c.	217	.5	.2
See also Wild rice.				
Rice cakes, brown rice	1 cake	35	.3	.1
Rice products, granulated–Packaged, used mainly as hot breakfast cereal, cooked	1 c.	130	.3	0
Rice products, puffed–Packaged, used mainly as ready-to-eat breakfast cereal plain, puffed rice	1 c.	29	trace	0
presweetened	1 c.	113	.2	0
presweetened, with cocoa	1 c.	138	.5	0
Rice pudding, prepared with 2% fat milk	½ c.	160	2.3	1.4

Cholesterol (mg)	Sodium (mg)	Carbohydrates (gm)		Protein (gm)
		Total	Fiber	
0	2	47.0	.?	4.5
0	29	7.3	.2	.7
0	3	28.8	0	2.3
0	6	trace	trace	.4
0	343	25.0	.1	1.9
0	273	31.7	.1	1.9
9	157	30.0	0	4.7

Food	Amount	Calories	Total Fat (gm)	Saturated Fat (gm)
Rolls and buns				
Home recipe Plain	1	119	3.0	–
Packaged Brown-and-serve–type rolls	1	70	1.0	0
Crescent, premade, refrigerated dough	1	80	3.0	1.0
Danish pastry, cheese	1 small	260	14.0	5.0
Frankfurter and hamburger rolls	1	110	2.0	0
Hard rolls, enriched	1	156	1.6	–
Raisin rolls or buns	1	280	8.0	2.0
Rutabagas, cooked	½ c. cubes	33	.2	trace

Cholesterol (mg)	Sodium (mg)	Carbohydrates (gm)		Protein (gm)
		Total	Fiber	
–	98	19.6	–	2.9
0	350	12.0	1.0	2.0
0	250	13.0	1.0	2.0
35	250	28.0	.1	4.0
0	210	20.0	1.0	4.0
–	313	29.9	–	4.9
30	230	49.0	1.0	5.0
0	17	7.3	1.0	1.1

Food	Amount	Calories	Total Fat (gm)	Saturated Fat (gm)
S				
Salad Dressings				
Commercial, low calorie, low fat				
Blue cheese	1 Tbsp.	40	4.0	1.0
French/Russian	1 Tbsp.	22	1.0	.1
Italian	1 Tbsp.	16	trace	.2
Ranch/Creamy Italian	1 Tbsp.	40	3.0	.3
Commercial, nonfat				
Blue cheese	1 Tbsp.	10	0	0
French/Russian	1 Tbsp.	15	0	0
Italian	1 Tbsp.	10	0	0
Ranch/Creamy Italian	1 Tbsp.	20	0	0
Commercial, regular				
Blue cheese	1 Tbsp.	78	8.0	1.5
French/Russian	1 Tbsp.	66	6.3	1.5

Cholesterol (mg)	Sodium (mg)	Carbohydrates (gm)		Protein (gm)
		Total	Fiber	
0	205	1.0	0	5
1	129	3.6	trace	trace
1	117	.7	trace	trace
0	155	2.5	0	0
0	135	2.0	0	0
0	110	3.5	0	0
0	145	1.0	0	0
0	135	4.5	0	0
—	—	1.1	trace	.7
—	210	2.7	.1	.1

Food	Amount	Calories	Total Fat (gm)	Saturated Fat (gm)
Salad Dressings Commercial, regular *(cont'd)* Italian	1 Tbsp.	69	7.1	1.0
Mayonnaise/ sandwich spread low fat	1 Tbsp.	25	1.0	0
nonfat	1 Tbsp.	10	0	0
regular	1 Tbsp.	99	11.0	1.2
Ranch/Creamy Italian	1 Tbsp.	85	9.0	1.5
Salmon, pink canned, solids with bone and liquid, no salt added	3 oz.	116	5.1	1.3
fresh, cooked	3 oz.	124	3.7	.6
Salt, table	1 tsp.	0	0	0
Sardines, Pacific, canned, in tomato sauce, drained	1	68	4.6	1.2

Cholesterol (mg)	Sodium (mg)	Carbohydrates (gm)		Protein (gm)
		Total	Fiber	
–	116	1.5	trace	.1
0	140	4.0	0	0
0	140	3.0	0	0
–	79	.4	0	.2
2.5	135	1.0	0	0
–	63	0	0	16.5
56	72	0	0	21.3
0	1720	0	0	0
23	159	0	trace	6.3

Food	Amount	Calories	Total Fat (gm)	Saturated Fat (gm)
Sauces Bearnaise, with milk, butter	¼ c.	172	16.8	10.3
Hollandaise, with milk, butter	¼ c.	173	16.8	10.3
White, with enriched flour, milk	¼ c.	57	3.2	1.5
See also Barbecue sauce.				
Sauerkraut, canned, solids and liquid	1 c.	48	.4	.1
Sausage Bratwurst, cooked	1 link	251	21.6	7.8
Brown-and-serve–type, browned	3 links	260	25.0	8.0
Italian, cooked	1 link	215	17.1	6.1
Knockwurst	1 link	205	18.5	6.8
Pepperoni	1 slice	27	2.4	.9
Polish-style	½ link	362	31.9	11.4

Cholesterol (mg)	Sodium (mg)	Carbohydrates (gm)		Protein (gm)
		Total	Fiber	
46	310	4.3	trace	2.1
46.3	278	4.4	trace	2.1
8.1	189	5.1	trace	3.2
0	1653	10.8	2.8	2.3
50	464	1.8	0	11.8
45	460	1.0	0	7.0
52	615	1.0	0	13.3
39	673	1.2	0	7.9
–	113	.2	0	1.2
78	973	1.8	0	15.7

Food	Amount	Calories	Total Fat (gm)	Saturated Fat (gm)
Sausage *(cont'd)* Pork, cooked	1 link	48	4.1	1.4
Scrapple	2 oz.	110	7.0	2.5
Turkey	1 link	140	8.0	2.0
Vienna, canned sausage	1	44	4.0	1.5
Scallops, raw	5 small	27	.2	trace
Sea bass, cooked	3 oz.	103	2.2	.5
Sesame seeds, dried	1 Tbsp.	47	4.4	.6
Shad, cooked	3 oz.	210	14.8	0
Shallots, raw	1 Tbsp.	7	trace	trace
Sherbert, orange	½ c.	135	1.9	1.2
Shrimp, cooked	4 large	90	1.0	.3
Snapper, cooked	3 oz.	106	1.4	.3
Soda. *See* **Beverages.**				

Cholesterol (mg)	Sodium (mg)	Carbohydrates (gm)		Protein (gm)
		Total	Fiber	
11	168	.1	0	2.6
45	440	6.0	0	5.0
70	760	2.0	0	18.0
8	151	.3	0	1.6
10	49	.7	0	5.1
44	73	0	0	19.7
0	3	.8	.2	2.1
0	54	0	0	18.1
0	1	1.6	.1	1.3
7	44	29.2	trace	1.1
177	204	0	0	19.0
39	48	0	0	21.9

Food	Amount	Calories	Total Fat (gm)	Saturated Fat (gm)
Soups				
Canned (prepared with water)				
Asparagus, cream of	1 c.	88	4.3	1.0
Beef broth, bouillon, and consommé	1 c.	18	.5	.3
Beef noodle	1 c.	85	3.3	1.3
Celery, cream of	1 c.	93	5.8	1.5
Chicken, cream of	1 c.	120	7.5	2.3
Chicken broth	1 c.	40	1.5	.5
Chicken gumbo	1 c.	58	1.5	.3
Chicken noodle	1 c.	78	2.5	.8
Chicken vegetable	1 c.	78	3.0	1.0
Chicken with rice	1 c.	63	2.0	.5
Clam chowder, Manhattan style	1 c.	80	2.3	.5
Lentil	1 c.	140	2.0	0

Cholesterol (mg)	Sodium (mg)	Carbohydrates (gm)		Protein (gm)
		Total	Fiber	
5	1005	11.0	.8	2.3
trace	815	trace	trace	2.8
5	975	9.3	trace	5.0
15	973	9.0	.5	1.8
10	1010	9.5	.1	3.5
0	795	1.0	trace	5.0
5	978	8.5	.3	2.8
8	1148	9.8	.3	4.3
10	980	9.0	.1	3.8
8	845	7.5	trace	3.8
3	1055	12.5	.5	2.3
0	750	22.0	7.0	9.0

Food	Amount	Calories	Total Fat (gm)	Saturated Fat (gm)
Soups (cont'd) Minestrone	1 c.	85	2.5	.5
Mushroom, cream of	1 c.	133	9.3	2.5
Onion, with water	1 c.	60	1.8	.3
Pea, green	1 c.	165	3.0	1.5
Pea, green, with ham	1 c.	188	4.3	1.8
Tomato	1 c.	88	2.0	.5
Vegetable	1 c.	75	2.0	.3
Dehydrated, packaged, undiluted Chicken noodle	1 packet	246	5.5	1.2
Onion	1 packet	113	2.3	.5
Vegetable beef	1 packet	246	5.1	2.6
Ready-to-serve (No water added) Vegetable, chunky	1 c.	128	3.8	.5

Cholesterol (mg)	Sodium (mg)	Carbohydrates (gm)		Protein (gm)
		Total	Fiber	
3	945	11.8	.8	4.5
3	1058	9.5	.5	2.5
0	1092	8.5	.5	4.0
0	988	26.5	.8	8.5
8	995	27.8	.8	10.3
0	893	17.0	.5	2.0
0	853	12.5	.5	2.3
10	5993	34.6	.3	13.7
2	3445	20.6	.9	4.5
6	4614	36.9	.7	13.5
0	1053	19.8	1.3	3.8

Food	Amount	Calories	Total Fat (gm)	Saturated Fat (gm)
Sour cream	1 Tbsp.	26	2.5	1.6
Soybean curd (tofu), regular, raw	½ c.	95	6.0	.9
Soybeans, (mature seeds) cooked	1 c.	74	4.1	.5
raw	1 c.	87	4.8	.6
Soy sauce	1 Tbsp.	10	1.5	trace
Spaghetti. *See* **Pasta.**				
Spanish rice, mix as prepared with tomatoes	1 c.	270	8.0	1.0
Spinach canned, drained	1 c.	49	1.1	.2
cooked	1 c.	41	.5	.1
frozen leaf, boiled, drained	1 c.	54	.4	trace
raw, chopped	1 c.	12	.2	trace

Cholesterol (mg)	Sodium (mg)	Carbohydrates (gm)		Protein (gm)
		Total	Fiber	
5	6	.5	0	.4
0	8.8	2.4	.1	10.1
0	9	5.9	1.8	7.7
0	10	6.9	1.6	9.4
0	1021	1.5	0	.9
0	1210	5.0	1.0	6.0
0	57	7.2	0	6.0
0	125	6.8	1.6	5.4
0	165	10.2	2.1	6.0
0	44	1.9	.5	1.6

Food	Amount	Calories	Total Fat (gm)	Saturated Fat (gm)
Squash				
Summer, all types cooked	1 c.	36	.5	.1
raw	1 c.	26	.3	.1
Winter, all types cooked	1 c.	78	1.3	.2
raw	½ med. squash	43	.2	.1
Zucchini cooked	1 c.	29	.1	trace
frozen, cooked	1 c.	43	.3	.1
raw	1 c.	18	.1	trace
Steak. *See* **Beef.**				
Strawberries fresh	1 c.	45	.6	trace
frozen, sliced, sweetened	½ c.	120	.2	trace
Sturgeon, cooked	3 oz.	113	4.3	1.0

Cholesterol (mg)	Sodium (mg)	Carbohydrates (gm)		Protein (gm)
		Total	Fiber	
0	2	7.7	1.1	1.6
0	3	5.7	.8	1.6
0	2	17.6	1.4	1.8
0	5	10.2	1.6	1.7
0	6	7.0	.9	1.1
0	5	9.0	1.5	3.0
0	4	3.8	.6	1.6
0	2	10.4	.7	.9
0	4	32.4	.8	.6
0	0	0	0	17.3

Food	Amount	Calories	Total Fat (gm)	Saturated Fat (gm)
Sugar Beet or cane brown	1 oz. packed	104	0	0
granulated	1 tsp.	15	0	0
powdered	1 oz. unsifted	58	trace	0
Maple	1 oz. (1 piece)	101	.1	0
Sunflower seed kernels, dried	1 oz.	163	14.2	1.5
Sweetbreads (thymus), beef, cooked	3 oz.	265	20.8	–
Sweet potatoes baked in skin	1 med.	118	.1	trace
candied	1 piece	144	3.5	1.5
Swordfish, cooked	3 oz.	129	4.3	1.2
Syrup Blends, cane and maple	1 Tbsp.	53	0	0

Cholesterol (mg)	Sodium (mg)	Carbohydrates (gm)		Protein (gm)
		Total	Fiber	
0	11	27.0	0	0
0	trace	4.0	0	0
0	trace	14.9	0	0
0	3	26.0	0	trace
0	1	5.4	1.2	6.5
245	97	0	0	18.3
0	0	27.9	.9	2.0
8	74	29.4	.4	.9
42	96	0	0	21.2
0	trace	13.7	0	0

Food	Amount	Calories	Total Fat (gm)	Saturated Fat (gm)
Syrup *(cont'd)* Corn, high fructose	1 Tbsp.	53	0	0
Maple	1 Tbsp.	52	trace	0
Syrup *(cont'd)* Maple, reduced calorie	1 Tbsp.	28	0	0

T

Food	Amount	Calories	Total Fat (gm)	Saturated Fat (gm)
Tangerine juice canned, sweetened	1 c.	125	.5	trace
frozen concentrate, diluted	1 c.	115	.3	trace
Tangerines, raw	1 med.	37	.2	trace
Tapioca pudding, prepared with 2% milk	½ c	149	2.4	1.4
Tartar sauce low calorie	2 Tbsp.	110	11.0	1.5
regular	2 Tbsp.	180	19.0	3.0

Cholesterol (mg)	Sodium (mg)	Carbohydrates (gm)		Protein (gm)
		Total	Fiber	
0	trace	14.3	0	0
0	2	13.4	0	0
0	31	6.5	0	0
0	3	30.0	.3	1.3
0	3	27.8	.8	1.0
0	1	9.3	.3	.5
9	174	28.1	0	4.1
0	85	3.0	0	0
15	270	2.0	0	0

Food	Amount	Calories	Total Fat (gm)	Saturated Fat (gm)
Tea, instant powder, prepared with water, unsweetened	1 c.	3	0	0
Tofu. *See* **Soybean curd.**				
Tomato catsup	1 packet	6	trace	trace
Tomato juice, canned, regular	8 oz.	21	.1	trace
Tomato paste, canned	¼ c.	53	.6	.1
Tomato purée, canned	1 c.	103	.3	.1
Tomato sauce canned, unseasoned	1 c.	75	.5	.1
Marinara, can or jar	1 c.	170	8.5	1.3
Tomatoes (ripe) canned, whole	1 c.	50	.5	.1
cooked	1 c.	68	1.0	.2

Cholesterol (mg)	Sodium (mg)	Carbohydrates (gm)		Protein (gm)
		Total	Fiber	
0	8	.5	0	0
0	71	1.6	.1	.1
0	451	5.3	.5	1.0
0	40	11.8	.6	2.4
0	50	25.0	2.0	4.3
trace	1512	18.0	1.8	3.3
0	1572	25.5	1.7	4.0
0	408	10.8	1.3	2.3
0	28	14.5	2.0	2.8

Food	Amount	Calories	Total Fat (gm)	Saturated Fat (gm)
Tomatoes *(cont'd)* raw	1 med.	26.2	.4	.1
Tongue, beef, cooked	3 oz.	236	17.3	7.4
Toppings Butterscotch or caramel	2 Tbsp.	105	trace	trace
Fruit	2 Tbsp.	106	trace	0
Trail mix	1 oz.	132	8.4	1.6
Trout, cooked	3 oz.	158	7.1	1.3
Tuna canned Chunk light, in oil	3 oz.	165	9.0	1.5
Chunk light, in water	3 oz.	90	.8	0
White, in oil	3 oz.	135	4.5	.8
White, in water	3 oz.	105	1.5	0
White, in water, drained, salted	3 oz.	113	2.1	.5

Cholesterol (mg)	Sodium (mg)	Carbohydrates (gm)		Protein (gm)
		Total	Fiber	
0	11	5.8	.9	1.1
89	50	.3	0	18.4
0	145	27.5	0	.6
0	9	27.6	.2	.1
0	65	12.8	.7	3.9
62	56	0	0	22.2
40	375	0	0	20.0
40	375	0	0	20.0
37	375	0	0	22.1
37	375	0	0	22.5
35	327	0	0	22.3

Food	Amount	Calories	Total Fat (gm)	Saturated Fat (gm)
Tuna *(cont'd)* fresh, Bluefin, cooked	3 oz.	153	5.3	1.3
Turkey dark meat, skinless, cooked	3 oz.	147	3.9	1.4
dark meat, with skin, cooked	3 oz.	165	6.5	1.9
light meat, skinless, cooked	3 oz.	127	1.1	.4
light meat, with skin, cooked	3 oz.	149	4.1	1.2
Turnip greens, cooked	1 c.	29	.3	.1
Turnips boiled, drained, diced	1 c.	30	.2	trace
raw	1 c.	36	.1	trace

V

Food	Amount	Calories	Total Fat (gm)	Saturated Fat (gm)
Veal Cubed for stew, lean only, cooked	3 oz.	157	3.6	1.1

Cholesterol (mg)	Sodium (mg)	Carbohydrates (gm)		Protein (gm)
		Total	Fiber	
41	42	0	0	24.9
102	72	0	0	26.2
106	69	0	0	25.2
78	51	0	0	27.5
86	52	0	0	26.2
0	41	6.3	.9	1.6
0	83	8.2	1.2	1.2
0	88	8.2	1.2	1.2
121	78	0	0	29.2

Food	Amount	Calories	Total Fat (gm)	Saturated Fat (gm)
Veal *(cont'd)* Ground, cooked	3 oz.	143	6.3	2.5
Loin, lean only, cooked	3 oz.	146	5.8	2.2
Sirloin, lean only, cooked	3 oz.	140	5.2	2.0
Vegetable juice cocktail, canned	8 oz.	23	.1	trace
Vegetable shortening	1 Tbsp.	113	12.8	3.2
Venison (deer), cooked	3 oz.	132	2.6	1.1
Vinegar, cider or white	½ oz.	2	0	0

W

Food	Amount	Calories	Total Fat (gm)	Saturated Fat (gm)
Waffles frozen	2	200	7.0	1.5
See also Pancakes and waffles.				
Walnuts, English or Persian, dried	1 oz.	183	17.7	1.6

Cholesterol (mg)	Sodium (mg)	Carbohydrates (gm)		Protein (gm)
		Total	Fiber	
86	69	0	0	20.3
88.	80	0	0	21.9
87	71	0	0	21.9
0	445	5.6	.2	.7
−	−	0	0	0
93	45	0	0	25.2
0	0	0	0	0
5.0	530	31.0	2.0	4.0
0	3	5.2	1.3	4.1

Food	Amount	Calories	Total Fat (gm)	Saturated Fat (gm)
Water chestnuts, Chinese, raw	½ c.	66	.1	0
Watercress, raw	½ c.	2	trace	trace
Watermelon	1 c.	51	.6	0
Wheat flour, white, all-purpose	1 c.	455	1.3	.3
Wheat germ, toasted	⅛ c.	50	1.4	.2
Wheat products— Packaged, used mainly as breakfast cereals cold, flakes	1 c.	103	.5	.1
cold, puffed, plain	1 c.	44	.1	0
cold, shredded, small biscuit	1 c.	156	.9	0
hot, creamy, instant, cooked, diluted	1 c.	160	.5	0
Whipped cream. *See* Cream.				

Cholesterol (mg)	Sodium (mg)	Carbohydrates (gm)		Protein (gm)
		Total	Fiber	
0	9	14.9	.5	.9
0	7	.2	.1	.4
0	3	11.4	.5	1.0
0	3	95.4	.4	12.9
0	1	6.5	.3	3.8
0	368	23.4	2.1	2.8
0	1	9.6	.4	1.8
0	4	34.7	4.0	4.8
0	8	32.8	3.0	4.5

Food	Amount	Calories	Total Fat (gm)	Saturated Fat (gm)
Whipped topping canned (pressurized)	1 Tbsp.	11	.9	.8
nondairy dessert topping	1 Tbsp.	13	1.0	.8
powdered, prepared with whole milk	1 Tbsp.	8	.5	.4
White sauce. *See* **Sauces.**				
Whitefish, cooked	3 oz.	143	6.3	1.0
Wild rice, cooked	1 c.	168	.5	.1
Wine. *See* **Beverages.**				

Y

Yams. *See* **Sweet potatoes.**				
Yogurt Fruit or flavored low fat	1 c.	255	2.8	1.8
nonfat, sugar free	1 c.	100	0	0

Cholesterol (mg)	Sodium (mg)	Carbohydrates (gm)		Protein (gm)
		Total	Fiber	
0	3	.6	0	trace
0	1	.9	0	.1
.4	3	.7	0	.1
64	54	0	0	20.4
0	5	35.6	.5	6.7
10	145	47.8	.3	11.0
5	140	17.0	0	9.0

Food	Amount	Calories	Total Fat (gm)	Saturated Fat (gm)
Yogurt *(cont'd)*				
Frozen				
hard, low fat	½ c.	160	2.0	1.0
soft-serve, vanilla	1 c.	227	8.0	4.9
Plain				
low fat	1 c.	143	3.5	2.3
nonfat	1 c.	127	.4	.3
whole milk	1 c.	138	7.4	4.8

Z

Zucchini. *See* Squash.			

Cholesterol (mg)	Sodium (mg)	Carbohydrates (gm)		Protein (gm)
		Total	Fiber	
5	6	32.0	6.0	4.0
3	124	34.6	.1	5.7
14	159	15.9	0	11.9
5	173	17.5	0	12.9
30	104	10.6	0	7.9

Suggested Weights for Adults

| Height[1] | Weight in pounds[2] | |
	19 to 34 years	35 years and over
5'0"	[3]97–128	108–138
5'1"	101–132	111–143
5'2"	104–137	115–148
5'3"	107–141	119–152
5'4"	111–146	122–157
5'5"	114–150	126–162
5'6"	118–155	130–167
5'7"	121–160	134–172
5'8"	125–164	138–178
5'9"	129–169	142–183
5'10"	132–174	146–188
5'11"	136–179	151–194
6'0"	140–184	155–199
6'1"	144–189	159–205
6'2"	148–195	164–210
6'3"	152–200	168–216
6'4"	156–205	173–222
6'5"	160–211	177–228
6'6"	164–216	182–234

[1] Without shoes.
[2] Without clothes.
[3] The higher weights in the ranges generally apply to men, who tend to have more muscle and bone; the lower weights more often apply to women, who have less muscle and bone.
Credit: National Research Council

Most of us eat more than we think, and more often. Sometimes we eat too much of one type of food, or not enough of another, creating a nutritional imbalance. Use this sample diary to record and evaluate

FIRST DAY

BREAKFAST

_____
_____
_____
_____
_____
_____

LUNCH

_____
_____
_____
_____
_____
_____

DINNER

_____
_____
_____
_____
_____
_____

SNACKS

_____
_____
_____
_____
_____

Daily Food Diary

your food intake or to set up your own meal plans. Remember to include beverages and items used in food preparation, such as oils and butter.

SECOND DAY

BREAKFAST

_____
_____
_____
_____
_____

LUNCH

_____
_____
_____
_____
_____

DINNER

_____
_____
_____
_____
_____

SNACKS

_____
_____
_____
_____
_____

10 Week Progress Chart for Weight Loss

Weigh yourself once a week (for example, every Monday if you begin your diet on a Monday), on the same scale, at the same time of day, wearing approximately the same amount of clothing. The first entry in the chart would come at the end of one full week of following your program.

Starting Weight _____ Goal Weight _____

Starting Date _____ Goal Date _____

	WEIGHT	**LOSS**
Week 1	_____	_____
Week 2	_____	_____
Week 3	_____	_____
Week 4	_____	_____
Week 5	_____	_____
Week 6	_____	_____
Week 7	_____	_____
Week 8	_____	_____
Week 9	_____	_____
Week 10	_____	_____

Abbreviations Used in This Book

approx.	approximately
av.	average
c.	cup(s)
choc.	chocolate
diam.	diameter
ea.	each
fl.	fluid
gm.	gram(s)
IU	international unit
lb.	pound
lg.	large
mcg	microgram(s)
med.	medium
min.	minute
mg	milligram(s)
oz.	ounce(s)
pkg.	package
serv.	serving(s)
Tbsp.	tablespoon(s)
tsp.	teaspoon(s)
w/	with
w/o	without

Guide to Equivalent Weights and Measures

By Volume (Liquid/Fluid)

1 cup = ½ pint = 8 fluid ounces = 237 milliliters
4 cups = 1 quart = 32 fluid ounces = 0.946 liter
4 quarts = 1 gallon = 128 fluid ounces = 3.785 liters

2 tablespoons = 1 fluid ounce = 30 milliliters
16 tablespoons = 1 cup = 237 milliliters
3 teaspoons = 1 tablespoon = 15 milliliters

⅓ cup = 5 tablespoons + 1 teaspoon
¾ cup = 12 tablespoons
⅞ cup = 14 tablespoons

By Weight (Avoirdupois)

1 ounce = 28.35 grams
3½ ounces = 100 grams
1 pound = 16 ounces = 453.6 grams
1 kilogram = 1000 grams = 2.2 pounds

Commercial Canned Goods

Av. Net Weight	Approx. Cups
8 oz.	1
10½–12 oz.	1¼
14–16 oz.	1¾
16–17 oz.	2
1 lb. 4 oz. (20 oz.)	2½
1 lb. 13 oz. (29 oz.)	3½

Estimating Portion Sizes

	uncooked amount	cooked yield
beans, dry	1 cup	2 cups
rice	1 cup	3 cups
spaghetti, dry	2 oz.	1 cup
chicken		
breast	1	3 oz.
thigh or drumstick	1	2 oz.
pork or lamb chop	1	3 oz.
ground beef, lean	4 oz.	3 oz.

Glossary

absorption, uptake of substances by a tissue, as of nutrients through the wall of the intestine.

additive, 1. a substance added directly to food during processing, as for preservation, coloring, or stabilization. **2.** something that becomes part of food or affects it as a result of packaging or processing, as debris or radiation.

agar or **agar-agar,** a gel prepared from the cell walls of various red algae, used in laboratories as a culture medium, in food processing as a thickener and stabilizer, and in industry as a filler, adhesive, etc.

albumin or **albumen,** any of a class of simple, sulfur-containing, water-soluble proteins that coagulate when heated, occurring in egg white, milk, blood, and other animal and vegetable tissues and secretions.

alimentary, 1. concerned with the function of nutrition; nutritive. **2.** pertaining to food.

alimentary canal, a tubular passage functioning in the digestion and absorption of food and the elimination of food residue, beginning at the mouth and terminating at the anus.

alkaloid, any of a large class of bitter-tasting, nitrogen-containing, alkaline ring compounds common in plants and including caffeine, morphine, nicotine, quinine, and strychnine.

allergen, any substance, usually a protein, that induces an allergic reaction in a particular individual.

alpha-tocopherol, VITAMIN E.

amino acid, any of a class of organic compounds that contains at least one amino group and one carboxyl group:, the alpha-amino acids are the building blocks from which proteins are constructed. See also ESSENTIAL AMINO ACID.

amylase, any of several digestive enzymes that break down starches.

analogue, a food made from vegetable matter, especially soybeans, that has been processed to taste and look like another food, as meat or dairy, and is used as a substitute for it.

anorectic also **anoretic, 1.** having no appetite. **2.** causing a loss of appetite. **3.** a substance, as a drug, causing loss of appetite.

anorexia nervosa, an eating disorder characterized by a fear of becoming fat, a distorted body image, and excessive dieting leading to emaciation.

anorexic, 1. a person suffering from anorexia or especially anorexia nervosa. **2.** ANORECTIC.

antinutrient, a substance that interferes with the utilization of one or more nutrients by the body, as oxalate and phytate, which prevent calcium absorption.

antioxidant, an enzyme or other organic substance, as vitamin E or beta carotene, capable of counteracting the damaging effects of oxidation in animal tissues.

Apgar score, a quantitative evaluation of the health of a newborn, rating breathing, heart rate, muscle tone, etc., on a scale of 1 to 10.

ascorbic acid, a white, crystalline, water-soluble vitamin occurring naturally in citrus fruits, green vegetables, etc., and also produced synthetically, essential for normal metabolism: used in the prevention and treatment of scurvy, and in wound-healing and tissue repair. Also called **vitamin C.**

aspartame, a white crystalline powder synthesized from amino acids, that is many times sweeter than sucrose and is used as a low-calorie sugar substitute.

assimilation, the conversion of absorbed food into the substance of the body.

autophagia also **autophagy,** the maintenance of bodily nutrition by the metabolic breakdown of some bodily tissues.

avitaminosis, any disease caused by a lack of vitamins.

balanced diet, a diet consisting of the proper quantities and proportions of foods needed to maintain health or growth.

bariatrics, (*used with a sing. v.*) a branch of medicine that deals with the control and treatment of obesity and allied diseases.

basal metabolic rate, the rate at which energy is expended while fasting and at rest, calculated as calories per hour per square meter of body surface. *Abbr.:* BMR

basal metabolism, the minimal amount of energy necessary to maintain respiration, circulation, and other vital body functions while fasting and at total rest.

B complex, VITAMIN B COMPLEX.

beta carotene, the most abundant of various isomers of carotene that can be converted by the body to vitamin A.

BHA, butylated hydroxyanisole: an antioxidant used to retard rancidity in products containing fat or oil.

BHT, butylated hydroxytoluene: an antioxidant used to retard rancidity in products containing fat or oil.

bioavailability, the extent to which a nutrient or medication can be used by the body.

bioflavonoid, any of a group of water-soluble yellow compounds, present in citrus fruits, rose hips, and other plants, that in mammals maintain the resistance of capillary walls to permeation and change of pressure. Also called **vitamin P.**

biogenic, 1. resulting from the activity of living organisms, as fermentation. **2.** necessary for the life process, as food and water.

biological value, the nutritional effectiveness of the protein in a given food, expressed as the percentage used by the body of either the total protein consumed or the digestible protein available.

biotin, a crystalline, water-soluble vitamin of the vitamin B complex, present in all living cells. Also called **vitamin H.**

BMR, basal metabolic rate.

bulimarexia, BULIMIA (def. 1).

bulimia, 1. Also called **bulimia**

nervosa. a habitual disturbance in eating behavior characterized by bouts of excessive eating followed by self-induced vomiting, purging with laxatives, strenuous exercise, or fasting. **2.** Also called **hyperphagia.** abnormally voracious appetite or unnaturally constant hunger.

caffeine, a white, crystalline, bitter alkaloid usually derived from coffee or tea, used medicinally as a stimulant.

caffeinism, chronic toxicity caused by excessive intake of caffeine, characterized by anxiety, irritability, palpitations, insomnia, and digestive disturbances.

calciferol, a fat-soluble, crystalline, unsaturated alcohol occurring in milk, fish-liver oils, etc., produced by ultraviolet irradiation of ergosterol and used as a dietary supplement, as in fortified milk. Also called **vitamin D₂.**

calcitriol, 1. a vitamin D compound derived from cholesterol, involved in the regulating and absorption of calcium. **2.** a preparation of this compound, used in the treatment of osteoporosis and bone fracture.

calcium, a silver-white divalent metal, combined in limestone, chalk, etc., occurring also in animals in bone, shell, etc. *Symbol:* Ca.

calcium propionate, a white, water-soluble powder used in bakery products to inhibit the growth of fungi.

calorie or **calory, 1. a.** Also called **gram calorie, small calorie.** an amount of heat exactly equal to 4,1840 joules. *Abbr.:* cal **b.** (*usually cap.*) KILOCALORIE. *Abbr.:* Cal **2. a.** a unit equal to the kilocalorie,

used to express the heat output of an organism and the energy value of food. **b.** the quantity of food capable of producing such an amount of energy.

calorifacient, (of foods) producing heat.

carbo, 1. carbohydrate. **2.** a food having a high carbohydrate content.

carbohydrate, any of a class of organic compounds composed of carbon, hydrogen, and oxygen, including starches and sugars, produced in green plants by photosynthesis: important source of food.

carbo-loading, the practice of eating large amounts of carbohydrates for a few days before competing in a strenuous athletic event, as a marathon, to provide energy reserves in the form of glycogen.

carotene also **carotin,** any of three yellow or orange fat-soluble pigments found in many plants, especially carrots, and transformed into vitamin A in the liver; provitamin A.

carrageenan or **carrageenin,** a colloidal substance extracted from seaweed used chiefly as an emulsifying and stabilizing ingredient in foods and pharmaceuticals.

casein, a protein precipitated from milk, as by rennet, and forming the basis of cheese.

CFNP, Community Food and Nutrition Programs.

Chinese-restaurant syndrome, a reaction, as headache or sweating, to monosodium glutamate, sometimes added to food in Chinese restaurants.

chlorine, a halogen element, a heavy, greenish-yellow, incombustible, water-soluble, poisonous gas that is highly irritating to the respiratory organs: used for water purification and in the manufacture of chemicals. *Symbol:* Cl

chlorophyll or **chlorophyl,** the green pigment of plant leaves and algae, essential to their production of carbohydrates by photosynthesis.

cholecalciferol, VITAMIN D_3.

cholesterol, a sterol abundant in animal fats, brain and nerve tissue, meat, and eggs, that functions in the body as a membrane constituent and as a precursor of steroid hormones and bile acids: high levels in the blood are associated with arteriosclerosis and gallstones.

choline, one of the B-complex vitamins, found in the lecithin of many plants and animals.

chromium, a lustrous metallic element used in alloy steels for hardness. *Symbol:* Cr

cobalamin also **cobalamine,** VITAMIN B_{12}.

code dating, the practice of placing a code indicating the date and site of packaging on certain products, as canned goods.

cod-liver oil, an oil extracted from the liver of cod and related fishes, used as a source of vitamins A and D.

collagen, a strongly fibrous protein that is abundant in bone, tendons, cartilage, and connective tissue, yielding gelatin when denatured by boiling.

complex carbohydrate, a carbohydrate, as sucrose or starch, that consists of two or more monosaccharide units. Compare SIMPLE CARBOHYDRATE.

copper, a metallic element having a reddish brown color: used as an electrical conductor and in the manufacture of alloys. *Symbol:* Cu

cyclamate, any of several chemical compounds used as a noncaloric sweetening agent in foods and beverages: banned by the FDA in 1970 as a possible carcinogen.

cystine, a crystalline amino acid occurring in most proteins, especially the keratins.

defibered, (of food) having little or no natural fiber, typically as the result of commercial refining or processing.

degerm, 1. to rid of germs. **2.** to remove the germ or embryo from (a kernel of grain), usually through milling.

dehydrate, 1. to lose an abnormal amount of water from the body. **2.** to free (fruit, vegetables, etc.) from moisture for preservation; dry.

dehydration, 1. the act or process of dehydrating. **2.** an abnormal loss of water from the body, especially from illness or physical exertion.

desiccate, to preserve (food) by removing moisture; dehydrate.

dextroglucose, DEXTROSE.

dextrose, the dextrorotatory form of glucose, occurring in fruits and in animal tissues and commercially obtainable from starch by acid hydrolysis.

DHA, docosahexaenoic acid: an omega-3 fatty acid present in fish oils.

diet, 1. food and drink considered in terms of qualities, composition, and effects on health. **2.** a particular selection of food, especially for improving a person's physical condition or to prevent or treat disease: *a low-fat diet.* **3.** such a selection or a limitation on the amount a person eats for reducing weight: *to go on a diet.* **4.** the foods habitually eaten by a particular person, animal, or group.

dietary fiber, FIBER.

dietetic, 1. pertaining to diet or to regulation of the use of food. **2.** prepared or suitable for special diets, especially those requiring a restricted sugar, salt, or caloric intake. **3. dietetics,** (*used with a sing. v.*) the science concerned with nutrition and food preparation.

dietitian or **dietician,** a person who is an expert in nutrition or dietetics.

digestion, 1. the process in the alimentary canal by which food is broken up physically, as by the action of the teeth, and chemically, as by the action of enzymes, and converted into a substance suitable for absorption and assimilation into the body. **2.** the function or power of digesting food.

digestive, 1. serving for or pertaining to digestion. **2.** promoting digestion. **3.** a substance promoting digestion.

digestive system, the system by which ingested food is acted upon by physical and chemical means to provide the body with absorbable nutrients and to excrete waste products: in mammals the system includes the alimentary canal extending from the mouth to the anus and the hormones and enzymes assisting in digestion.

D.R.V., (on food labels) Daily Reference Value: the amount of nutrients appropriate for one day.

dyspepsia also **dyspepsy,** deranged or impaired digestion; indigestion (opposed to *eupepsia*).

dyspeptic, 1. pertaining to, subject to, or suffering from dyspepsia. **2.** a person subject to or suffering from dyspepsia.

dystrophy also **dystrophia,** faulty or inadequate nutrition or development.

EDTA, ethylenediaminetetraacetic acid: a colorless compound capable of chelating a variety of divalent metal cations: used in food preservation, as an anticoagulant, and in the treatment of heavy-metal poisonings.

empty calorie, a calorie whose food source has little or no nutritional value.

enrich, 1. to restore to (a food) a nutrient lost in processing. **2.** to add vitamins and minerals to (food) to enhance its nutritive value.

enzyme, any of various proteins, as pepsin and amylase, originating from living cells and capable of producing certain chemical changes in organic substances by catalytic action, as in digestion.

EPA, eicosapentaenoic acid: an omega-3 fatty acid present in fish oils.

esophagus, a muscular tube for the passage of food from the pharynx to the stomach; gullet.

essential amino acid, any amino acid that is required for life and growth but is not produced in the body, or is produced in insufficient amounts, and must be supplied by protein in the diet.

eupepsia, good digestion (opposed to *dyspepsia*).

eutrophy, healthy or adequate nutrition or development.

expiration date, the last date that a product, as food, should be used before it is considered spoiled or ineffective, usually specified on the label or package.

extender, a substance added to another substance, as to food, to increase its volume or bulk.

fat, 1. any of several oily substances that are the chief component of animal adipose tissue and many plant seeds. **2.** animal tissue containing much fat. **3.** obesity; corpulence.

fat-soluble, capable of dissolving in oil or fats.

fatty acid, any of a class of organic acids consisting of a long hydrocarbon chain ending in a carboxyl group that bonds to glycerol to form a fat.

FDA, Food and Drug Administration.

FD&C color, any of the synthetic pigments and dyes that are approved by the FDA for use in foods, drugs, and cosmetics.

fiber, the structural parts of plants, as cellulose, pectin, and lignin, that are wholly or partly indigestible, acting to increase intestinal bulk and peristalsis.

fish protein concentrate, an odorless and tasteless high-protein food additive made from ground fish and suitable for human consumption. *Abbr.:* FPC

fluoride, 1. a salt of hydrofluoric acid consisting of two elements, one of which is fluorine, as sodium fluoride. **2.** a compound containing fluorine.

fluorine, the most reactive nonmetallic element, a pale yellow, corrosive, toxic gas that occurs combined in minerals and is found naturally in bones and teeth. *Symbol:* F

folate, FOLIC ACID.

folic acid, a water-soluble vitamin that is converted to a coenzyme essential to purine and thymine biosynthesis: deficiency causes a form of anemia.

food additive, additive (def. 1).

food poisoning, 1. any illness, as salmonellosis or botulism, caused by eating food contaminated with bacterial toxins and typically marked by severe intestinal symptoms, as diarrhea, vomiting, and cramps. **2.** any illness caused by eating poisonous mushrooms, plants, fish, etc., or food containing chemical contaminants.

food science, the study of the nature of foods and the changes that occur in them naturally and as a result of handling and processing.

formula, 1. a recipe or prescription. **2.** a special nutritive mixture, especially of milk or milk substitute with other ingredients, in prescribed proportions for feeding a baby.

fortify, to add one or more ingredients to (a food) to increase its nutritional content.

freshness date, the last date, usually specified on the label or packaging, that a food, as bread, is considered fresh, although it may be sold, ordinarily at reduced prices, or eaten after that date.

fructose, a yellowish to white, crystalline, water-soluble, levorotatory ketose sugar sweeter than sucrose, occurring in invert sugar, honey, and a great many fruits: used in foodstuffs and in medicine chiefly in solution as an intravenous nutrient. Also called **levulose, fruit sugar.**

fruitarian, a person whose diet consists chiefly of fruit.

gliadin, a simple protein of cereal grains that imparts elastic properties to flour: used as a nutrient in high-protein diets.

glucose, a simple sugar that is a product of photosynthesis and is the principal source of energy for all living organisms: concentrated in fruits and honey or readily obtainable from starch, other carbohydrates, or glycogen.

gluten, a grayish, sticky component of wheat flour and other grain flours, composed mainly of the proteins gliadin and glutenin.

glutenin, a simple protein of cereal grains that imparts adhesive properties to flour.

glycerin also **glycerine,** GLYCEROL.

glycerol, a colorless liquid used as a sweetener and preservative, and in suppositories and skin emollients.

glycine, a sweet crystalline solid, the simplest amino acid, present in most proteins. *Abbr.:* Gly; *Symbol:* G

glycogen, a polysaccharide composed of glucose isomers, that is the principal carbohydrate stored by the animal body and is readily converted to glucose when needed for energy use.

gorp, a mixture of nuts, raisins, dried fruits, seeds, or the like eaten as a high-energy snack, as by hikers and climbers.

granola, a breakfast food consisting of rolled oats, brown sugar, nuts, dried fruit, etc., usually served with milk.

GRAS, generally recognized as safe: a status label assigned by the FDA to a listing of substances (GRAS list) not known to be hazardous to health.

growth factor, any of various proteins that promote the growth, organization, and maintenance of cells and tissues.

growth hormone, any substance that stimulates or controls the growth of an organism, especially a species-specific hormone, as the human hormone somatotropin.

HDL, high-density lipoprotein.

health food, any natural food popularly believed to promote or sustain good health, as through its vital nutrients.

high-density lipoprotein, a circulating lipoprotein that picks up cholesterol in the arteries and deposits it in the liver for reprocessing or excretion. *Abbr.:* HDL

holism, an approach to healing or health care, often involving therapies outside the mainstream of medicine, in which isolated symptoms or conditions are considered secondary to one's total physical and psychological state.

holistic, 1. incorporating the concept of holism in theory or practice. **2.** identifying with principles of holism in a system of therapeutics, especially one considered outside the mainstream of scientific medicine, as naturopathy or chiropractic, and usually involving nutritional measures.

hormone, 1. any of various internally secreted compounds that are formed in endocrine glands and that affect the functions of specifically receptive organs or tissues when transported to them by the body fluids. **2.** a synthetic substance that acts like such a compound when introduced into the body.

human growth hormone, SO-MATOTROPIN. *Abbr.:* hGH

HVP or **H.V.P.,** HYDROLYZED VEGETABLE PROTEIN.

hydrogenate, to combine or treat with hydrogen, esp. to add it to (an unsaturated organic compound).

hydrolyzed vegetable protein, a vegetable protein broken down into amino acids and used as a food additive to enhance flavor.

hyperphagia, BULIMIA (def. 2).

inositol, a compound occurring in animal tissue, plants, and many seeds, and functioning as a growth factor.

insulin, 1. a hormone, produced by the beta cells of the islets of Langerhans of the pancreas, that regulates the metabolism of glucose and other nutrients. **2.** any of several commercial preparations of this substance, each absorbed into the body at a particular rate: used for treating diabetes.

intestinal bypass, the surgical circumvention of a diseased portion of the intestine; also sometimes used to reduce nutrient absorption in morbidly obese patients.

intestine, 1. Usually, **intestines.** the lower part of the alimentary canal, extending from the pylorus to the anus. **2.** Also called **small intestine.** the narrow, longer part of the intestines, comprising the duodenum, jejunum, and ileum, that serves to digest and absorb nutrients. **3.** Also called **large intestine.** the broad, shorter part of the intestines, comprising the cecum, colon, and rectum, that absorbs water from and eliminates the residues of digestion.

invert sugar, a mixture of the dextrorotatory forms of glucose and fructose formed naturally in fruits and produced artificially by treating cane sugar with acids.

iodine, a nonmetallic halogen element occurring as a grayish-black crystalline solid that sublimes to a dense violet vapor when heated: used as an antiseptic and as a nutritional supplement. *Symbol:* I

iron, 1. a ductile, malleable, silver-white metallic element, used in its impure carbon-containing forms for making tools, implements, machinery, etc. *Symbol:* Fe **2.** a preparation of iron or containing iron, used chiefly in the treatment of anemia.

isoleucine, a crystalline amino acid occurring in proteins, that is essential to the nutrition of humans and animals. *Abbr.:* Ile; *Symbol:* I

IV, an apparatus for intravenous delivery of electrolyte solutions, medicines, and nutrients.

junk food, food, as potato chips or candy, that is high in calories but of little nutritional value.

kwashiorkor, a disease, chiefly of children, caused by severe protein and vitamin deficiency and characterized by retarded growth, potbelly, and anemia.

lactarian, lactovegetarian (def. 1).

lactase, an enzyme capable of breaking down lactose into glucose and galactose.

lactation, 1. the secretion of milk. **2.** the period of milk production.

lactobacillus, any of various anaerobic bacteria capable of breaking down carbohydrates to form lactic acid: cultured for use in fermenting milk into yogurt or other milk products.

lactogenic, stimulating lactation.

lacto-ovo-vegetarian, 1. Also called **lactovarian, ovolactarian, ovo-lacto-vegetarian.** a vegetarian whose diet includes dairy products and eggs. **2.** pertaining to or maintaining a vegetarian diet that includes dairy products and eggs.

lactose, a disaccharide present in milk, that upon hydrolysis yields glucose and galactose.

lactovegetarian, 1. Also called **lactarian.** a vegetarian whose diet includes dairy products. **2.** pertaining to or maintaining a vegetarian diet that includes dairy products.

LDL, low-density lipoprotein.

lecithin, any of a group of phospholipids, containing choline and fatty acids, that are a component of cell membranes and are abundant in nerve tissue and egg yolk.

leucine, a white, crystalline, water-soluble amino acid obtained by the decomposition of proteins and made synthetically: essential in the nutrition of humans and animals. *Abbr.*: Leu; *Symbol*: L

levulose, FRUCTOSE.

lipase, any of a class of enzymes that break down fats, produced by the liver, pancreas, and other digestive organs or by certain plants.

liquid protein, an amino acid hydrosol used in weight-reduction programs as a substitute for all or some meals: generally regarded as hazardous to health because of low nutritional content and recommended for controlled use only under medical supervision.

low-density lipoprotein, a plasma protein that is the major carrier of cholesterol in the blood, with high levels being associated with atherosclerosis. *Abbr.*: LDL

lysine, a crystalline, basic, amino acid produced chiefly from many proteins by hydrolysis, essential in the nutrition of humans and animals. *Abbr.*: Lys; *Symbol*: K

macrobiotic, of or pertaining to macrobiotics.

macrobiotics, (*used with a sing. v.*) a program emphasizing harmony with nature, especially through a restricted, primarily vegetarian diet.

macromineral, any mineral required in the diet in relatively large amounts, especially calcium, iron, magnesium, phosphorus, potassium, and zinc.

macronutrient, any of the nutritional components required in relatively large amounts: protein, carbohydrate, fat, and the essential minerals.

magnesium, a ductile, silver-white metallic element that burns with a dazzling light. *Symbol*: Mg

malabsorption, faulty absorption of nutritive material from the intestine.

malassimilation, imperfect incorporation of nutrients into body tissue.

malnourished, poorly or improperly nourished; suffering from malnutrition.

malnutrition, lack of proper nutrition; inadequate or unbalanced nutrition.

maltose, a white, crystalline, water-soluble sugar formed by the action of diastase, especially from malt, on starch: used chiefly as a nutrient or sweetener, and in culture media. Also called **malt sugar.**

megavitamin, of, pertaining to, or using very large amounts of vitamins: *megavitamin therapy.*

menadione, a synthetic yellow crystalline powder, insoluble in water, used as a vitamin K supplement. Also called **vitamin K$_3$**.

metabolism, the sum of the physical and chemical processes in an organism by which its substance is produced, maintained, and destroyed, and by which energy is made available. Compare ANABOLISM, CATABOLISM.

metabolize, 1. to subject to or change by metabolism. **2.** to effect metabolism.

micronutrient, an essential nutrient, as a trace mineral, that is required in minute amounts.

mineral, any of the inorganic elements, as calcium, chromium, iron, magnesium, potassium, selenium, or sodium, that are essential to the functioning of the human body and are obtained from foods.

monosodium glutamate, a white, crystalline, water-soluble powder used to intensify the flavor of foods. Also called **MSG**. See also CHINESE-RESTAURANT SYNDROME.

monounsaturate, a monounsaturated fat or fatty acid, as olive oil.

monounsaturated, (of an organic compound) lacking a hydrogen bond at one point on the carbon chain.

MSG, monosodium glutamate.

multivitamin, 1. containing or consisting of several vitamins. **2.** a compound of several vitamins.

natural, having undergone little or no processing and containing no chemical additives.

naturopathy, a method of treat-

ing disease that employs no surgery or synthetic drugs but uses fasting, special diets, massage, etc., to assist the natural healing processes.

neurotrophic, of or pertaining to the effect of nerves on the nutritive processes.

neurotrophy, the influence of the nerves on the nutrition and maintenance of body tissue.

niacin, NICOTINIC ACID.

nicotinamide, a soluble crystal amide of nicotinic acid that is a component of the vitamin B complex and is present in most foods. Also called **niacinamide**.

nicotinic acid, a crystalline acid that is a component of the vitamin B complex, occurring in animal products, yeast, etc. Also called **niacin, vitamin B$_3$**.

nitrite, SODIUM NITRITE.

nitrogen, a colorless, odorless, gaseous element that constitutes about four-fifths of the volume of the atmosphere and is present in combined form in animal and vegetable tissues, especially in proteins. *Symbol:* N

nourish, to sustain with food or nutriment; supply with what is necessary for life, health, and growth.

nourishment, something that nourishes; food, nutriment, or sustenance.

NutraSweet, *Trademark.* a brand of aspartame used in a low-calorie sweetener and in other processed foods, as soft drinks.

nutrient, 1. nourishing; providing nourishment or nutriment. **2.** containing or conveying nutriment, as solutions or vessels of the body. **3.** a nutrient substance.

nutrient-dense, (of food) relatively rich in nutrients for the number of calories contained.

nutriment, 1. any substance that, taken into a living organism, serves to sustain it, promoting growth, replacing loss, and providing energy. **2.** anything that nourishes; nourishment; food.

nutrition, 1. the study or science of the dietary requirements of humans and animals for proper health and development. **2.** the process by which organisms take in and utilize food material. **3.** food; nutriment.

nutritionist, a person who is trained or expert in the science of nutrition.

nutritious, providing nourishment, especially to a high degree; nourishing; healthful.

nutritive, 1. serving to nourish; nutritious. **2.** of, pertaining to, or concerned with nutrition. **3.** an item of nourishing food.

omega-3 fatty acid, a fatty acid found especially in fish oil and valuable in reducing cholesterol levels in the blood.

open dating, the practice of putting a freshness date on food packages.

organic, pertaining to, involving, or grown with fertilizers or pesticides of animal or vegetable origin, as distinguished from manufactured chemicals: *organic farming; organic fruits.*

overnutrition, the excessive intake of food, especially in unbalanced proportions.

ovolactarian, lacto-ovo-vegetarian.

ovo-lacto-vegetarian, lacto-ovo-vegetarian.

pancreas, a large compound gland, situated near the stomach, that secretes digestive enzymes into the intestine and glucagon and insulin into the bloodstream.

pancreatic juice, a colorless alkaline fluid secreted by the pancreas, containing enzymes that break down protein, fat, and starch.

pancreatin, a mixture of the pancreatic enzymes trypsin, amylase, and lipase, used to promote digestion.

pantothenic acid, a hydroxy acid that is a component of the vitamin B complex, abundant in liver, yeast, and bran.

pepsin, 1. an enzyme, produced in the stomach, that splits proteins into proteoses and peptones. **2.** a commercial preparation containing pepsin, obtained from hog stomachs, used chiefly as a digestive and as a ferment in making cheese.

peptic, 1. pertaining to or associated with digestion; digestive. **2.** promoting digestion.

PGA, FOLIC ACID. [*p*(*teroyl*) + *g*(*lutamic*) *a*(*cid*)]

phenmetrazine, a compound used chiefly to control the appetite in the treatment of obesity.

phenylalanine, a crystalline, water-soluble, essential amino acid necessary to the nutrition of humans and most animals, occurring in egg white and skim milk. *Abbr.:* Phe; *Symbol:* F

phosphorus, a nonmetallic element existing in yellow, red, and black allotropic forms and an essential constituent of plant and animal tissue: used, in combined form, in matches and fertilizers. *Symbol:* P

phylloquinone, VITAMIN K_1.

phytonadione, VITAMIN K_1.

polyunsaturate, a type of fat found in vegetable oils that tends to lower cholesterol levels in the blood when substituted for saturated fats.

polyunsaturated, of or noting a class of animal or vegetable fats, especially plant oils, whose molecules consist of carbon chains with many double bonds unsaturated by hydrogen atoms and that are associated with a low cholesterol content of the blood.

potassium, a silvery white metallic element: essential in metabolism and for maintenance of normal fluid balance. *Symbol:* K

predigest, to treat (food) by an artificial process analogous to digestion so that, when taken into the body, it is more easily digestible.

preservative, a chemical substance used to preserve foods or other organic materials from decomposition or fermentation.

protein, 1. any of numerous organic molecules constituting a large portion of the mass of every life form, composed of 20 or more amino acids linked in one or more long chains, the final shape and other properties of each protein being determined by the side chains of the amino acids and their chemical attachments. **2.** plant or animal tissue rich in such molecules, considered as a food source.

provitamin, a substance that an organism can transform into a vitamin, as carotene, which is converted to vitamin A in the liver.

provitamin A, CAROTENE.

PUFA, polyunsatured fatty acid.

pull date, the last date on which perishable food should be sold, usually established with some allowance for home storage under refrigeration. Also called **sell date.** Compare SHELF LIFE.

purine, a white, crystalline compound from which is derived a group of compounds including uric acid, xanthine, and caffeine.

pyridoxine also **pyridoxin,** a derivative of pyridine, required for the formation of hemoglobin and the prevention of pellagra; vitamin B_6.

recommended dietary allowance, the amount of an essential nutrient, as a vitamin or mineral, that has been established by the Food and Nutrition Board of the National Academy of Sciences as adequate to meet the average daily nutritional needs of most healthy persons according to age group and sex. *Abbr.:* RDA Compare U.S. RDA.

Red No. 2, an artificial red dye used in foods, drugs, and cosmetics: banned by the FDA in 1976 as a possible carcinogen.

registered dietitian, a person who has fulfilled all the educational and examination requirements of the American Dietetic Association for recognition as a qualified nutrition specialist.

retinol, VITAMIN A.

riboflavin, a vitamin B complex factor essential for growth, occurring as a yellow crystalline compound abundant in milk, meat, eggs, and leafy vegetables and produced synthetically. Also called **vitamin B_2.**

saccharin, a white, crystalline, slightly water-soluble powder produced synthetically, which in dilute solution is 500 times as sweet as sugar: its soluble sodium salt is used as a noncaloric sugar substitute in the manufacture of syrups, foods, and beverages.

saturate, a saturated fat or fatty acid.

saturated fat, any animal or vegetable fat, abundant in fatty meats, dairy products, coconut oil, and palm oil, tending to raise cholesterol levels in the blood.

sea salt, table salt produced through the evaporation of seawater.

selenium, a nonmetallic element with an electrical resistance that varies under the influence of light. *Symbol:* Se

sell date, PULL DATE.

simple carbohydrate, a carbohydrate, as glucose, that consists of a single monosaccharide unit. Compare COMPLEX CARBOHYDRATE.

sitology, the branch of medicine dealing with nutrition and dietetics.

sodium, 1. a soft, silver-white, chemically active metallic element that occurs naturally only in combination: a necessary element in the body for the maintenance of normal fluid balance and other physiological functions. *Symbol:* NA **2.** any salt of sodium, as sodium chloride or sodium bicarbonate.

sodium nitrate, a crystalline, water-soluble compound that occurs naturally as soda niter: used in fertilizers, explosives, and glass, and as a color fixative in processed meats.

sodium nitrite, a yellowish or white crystalline compound used as a color fixative and in food as a flavoring and preservative.

somatotropin, a polypeptide growth hormone of humans, secreted by the anterior pituitary gland. Also called **human growth hormone.**

sorbitol, a sugar alcohol naturally occurring in many fruits or synthesized, used as a sugar substitute and in the manufacture of vitamin C.

stabilizer, any of various substances added to foods, chemical compounds, etc., to prevent deterioration, the breaking down of an emulsion, or the loss of desirable properties.

starch blocker or **starchblock,** a substance ingested in the belief that it inhibits the body's ability to metabolize starch and thereby promotes weight loss: declared illegal in the U.S. by the FDA.

sugar, 1. a sweet, crystalline substance obtained from the juice or sap of many plants, especially commercially from sugarcane and the sugar beet; sucrose. **2.** any other plant or animal substance of the same class of carbohydrates, as fructose or glucose.

sulfite, any sulfite-containing compound, especially one that is used in foods or drug products as a preservative.

TDN or **t.d.n.,** totally digestible nutrients.

thiamine also **thiamin,** a crystalline, water-soluble vitamin-B compound abundant in liver, legumes, and cereal grains. Also called **vitamin B**$_1$.

tocopherol, any of several oils that constitute vitamin E.

total parenteral nutrition, intravenous administration of a solution of essential nutrients to patients unable to ingest food.

TPN, total parenteral nutrition.

trophic, of or pertaining to nutrition; involving nutritive processes: *a trophic disease.*

TVP, *Trademark.* a brand of textured soy protein having various commercial uses as a meat substitute or extender.

undernourished, not nourished with sufficient or proper food to maintain health or normal growth.

undernutrition, nutritional deficiency resulting from lack of food or from the inability of the body to convert or absorb it.

uric acid, a compound present in urine in small amounts as the product of the metabolism of purines.

U.S. RDA, United States recommended daily allowance: the daily amount of a protein, vitamin, or mineral that the FDA has established as sufficient to maintain the nutritional health of persons in various age groups and categories, derived from the RDA developed by the Food and Nutrition Board of the National Academy of Sciences and used in the nutritional labeling of food. Compare RECOMMENDED DIETARY ALLOWANCE.

vegan, a vegetarian who omits all animal products from the diet.

vegetarian, 1. a person who does not eat meat, fish, fowl, or, in some cases, any food derived from animals. **2.** of or pertaining to vegetarianism or vegetarians.

vegetarianism, the practices or beliefs of a vegetarian.

vitamin, any of a group of organic substances essential in small quantities to normal metabolism, found in minute amounts in natural foodstuffs and also produced synthetically: deficiencies of vitamins produce specific disorders.

vitamin A, a yellow, fat-soluble alcohol obtained from carotene and occurring in green and yellow vegetables, egg yolk, etc.: essential to growth, the protection of epithelial tissue, and the prevention of night blindness. Also called **vitamin A₁, retinol.**

vitamin A₂, a yellow oil similar to vitamin A, obtained from fish liver.

vitamin B₁, THIAMINE.

vitamin B₂, RIBOFLAVIN.

vitamin B₃, NICOTINIC ACID.

vitamin B₆, PYRIDOXINE.

vitamin B₁₂, a complex water-soluble solid obtained from liver, milk, eggs, fish, oysters, and clams: a deficiency causes pernicious anemia and disorders of the nervous system. Also called **cobalamin.**

vitamin B complex, an important group of water-soluble vitamins containing vitamin B₁, vitamin B₂, etc.

vitamin C, ASCORBIC ACID.

vitamin D, any of the several fat-soluble vitamins occurring in milk and fish-liver oils, especially cod and halibut: essential for the formation of normal bones and teeth.

vitamin D₁, a form of vitamin D obtained by ultraviolet irradiation of ergosterol.

vitamin D₂, CALCIFEROL.

vitamin D₃, a form of vitamin D occurring in fish-liver oils, that differs from vitamin D₂ by slight structural differences in the molecule. Also called **cholecalciferol.**

vitamin E, a pale yellow viscous fluid, abundant in vegetable oils, whole-grain cereals, butter, and eggs, and important as an antioxidant in the deactivation of free radicals and in maintenance of the body's cell membranes: deficiency is rare. Also called **alpha-tocopherol.** Compare TOCOPHEROL.

vitamin G, RIBOFLAVIN.

vitamin H, BIOTIN.

vitamin K$_1$, a yellowish, oily, viscous liquid that occurs in leafy vegetables, rice, bran, and hog liver or is obtained especially from alfalfa or putrefied sardine meat or synthesized and that promotes blood clotting by increasing the prothrombin content of the blood. Also called **phylloquinone, phytonadione.**

vitamin K$_2$, a light yellow, crystalline solid having properties similar to those of vitamin K$_1$.

vitamin K$_3$, MENADIONE.

vitamin M, FOLIC ACID.

vitamin P, BIOFLAVONOID.

water-soluble, capable of dissolving in water.

xanthan, a gum produced by bacterial fermentation and used commercially as a binder or food stabilizer. Also called **xanthan gum.**

xanthine, a crystalline, nitrogenous compound related to uric acid, occurring in urine, blood, and certain animal and vegetable tissues.

yeast, 1. any of various small, single-celled fungi that reproduce by fission or budding and are capable of fermenting carbohydrates into alcohol and carbon dioxide. **2.** any of several yeasts used in brewing alcoholic beverages, as a leaven in baking breads, and in pharmacology as a source of vitamins and proteins.

Yellow No. 5, a yellow dye used in food, drugs, cosmetics, and other products: required by FDA regulations to be identified on food labels because of possible allergic reactions.

zinc, a ductile, bluish white metallic element: essential in minute quantities for physiological functioning. *Symbol:* Zn